DOCTOR SEBI:

The Real 7 Days Healing Journey with a Balanced Alkaline Plant-Based Diet. 200 Easy and Tasty Recipes, Approved Food List, Detox Smoothies to Lose Weight and Boost Your Health.

Lauren Hill

Table of Contents

INTRODUCTION

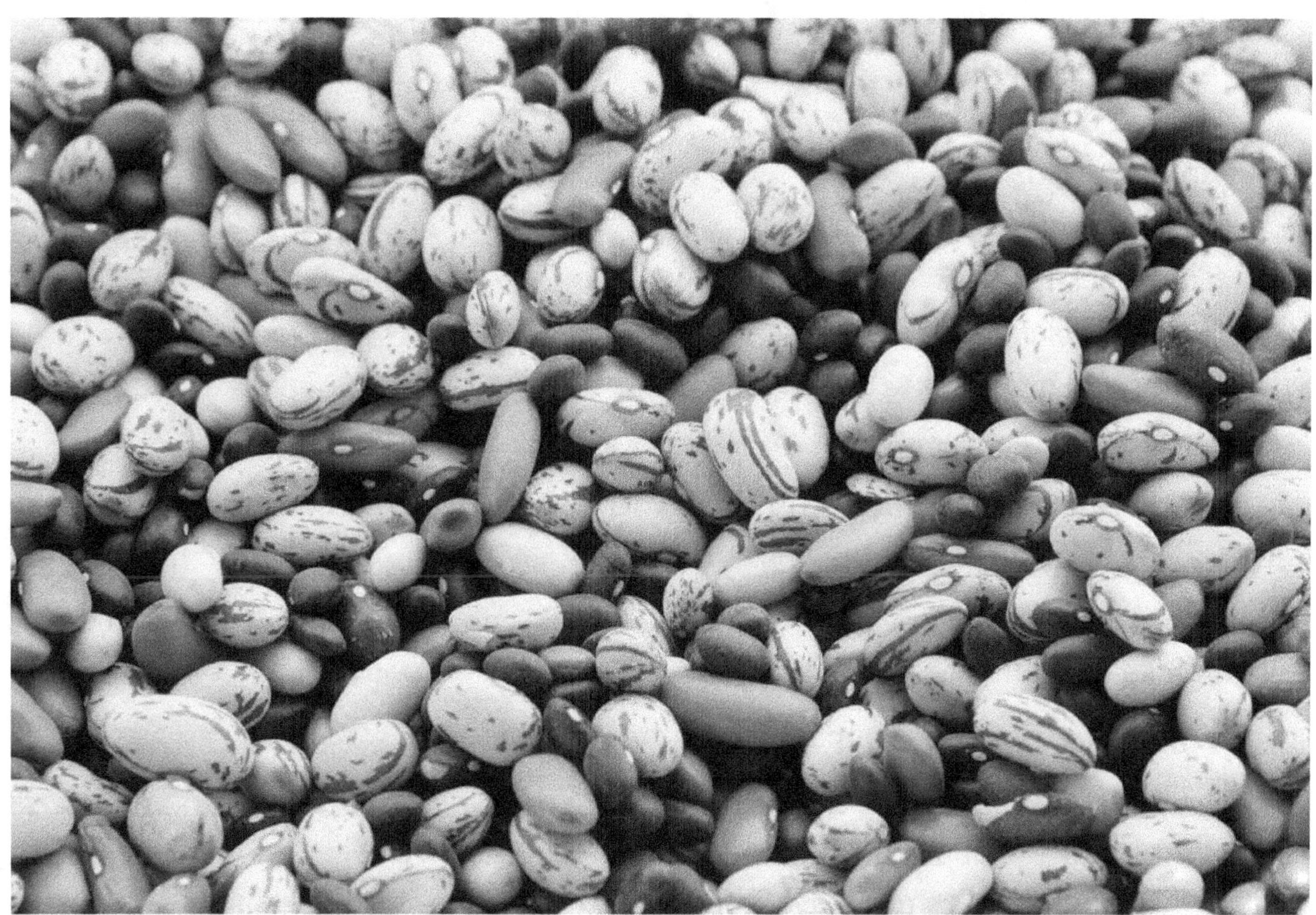

The Alkaline Diet and Intracellular Cleansing

The Alkaline Diet is a way of eating that balances your pH levels by choosing the right foods, mostly alkaline based, to maintain good health. Becoming familiar with the right types of food items to include in your diet is as simple as learning whether each item on your grocery list is alkaline or acidic.

Before your next trip to the supermarket, review the list of items or write down the foods you usually include on a typical shopping trip. For example, your list may contain the following items:

- Milk (2L)
- Bread
- Yogurt
- Apples (1 bag)
- Butter
- Ground beef (2 lbs.)
- Breakfast sausage
- Potatoes (1 bag)
- Eggs (1 dozen)
- Spinach (frozen)
- Case of pop/soda (12 cans)
- Tomatoes
- Mayonnaise
- Granola bars (1 box)
- Garlic

In total, there are fifteen items on this grocery list. How many of them are acidic versus alkaline? The results may be surprising:

<u>Acidic:</u> milk, bread, yogurt, butter, ground beef, breakfast sausage, eggs, pop/soda, mayonnaise, granola bars

<u>Alkaline:</u> apples, potatoes, spinach, tomatoes, garlic

Two-thirds of these items are acidic, while the remaining is alkaline. It is important to note that all the alkaline foods on this list are vegetables and fruits. In general, nearly all fruits and vegetables are alkaline-based, which makes a plant-based diet a good foundation to build an alkaline diet. The key is a balance, even with acidic foods as part of your regular diet, by increasing the alkaline content significantly over time. This will have a major improvement in your health in many ways.

Below is an idea of how your shopping list might look if you choose to follow Dr. Sebi's diet.

Fruit

Add any of the following Dr. Sebi-approved fruits to your shopping list:

- Bananas
- Apples
- Currants
- Berries
- Cantaloupe
- Dates
- Figs
- Tamarind
- Papayas
- Oranges
- Pears
- Plums
- Melons
- Peaches
- Cherries
- Grapes
- Limes
- Mangoes
- Raisins
- Prunes

Grains

Add any of the following Dr. Sebi-approved grains to your shopping list:

- Wild rice
- Kamut
- Amaranth
- Spelt
- Rye
- Quinoa
- Tef

- Fonio

Vegetables

Add any of the following Dr. Sebi-approved vegetables to your shopping list

- Bell peppers
- Amaranth
- Avocados
- Arame
- Dandelion greens
- Nori
- Lettuce (excluding iceberg)
- Mushrooms
- Garbanzo beans
- Kale
- Chayote
- Onions
- Tomatillo
- Olives
- Okra
- Squash
- Wild arugula
- Zucchini
- Wakame
- Watercress
- Turnip greens

Chapter 1

EXCESS MUCUS IN THE BODY

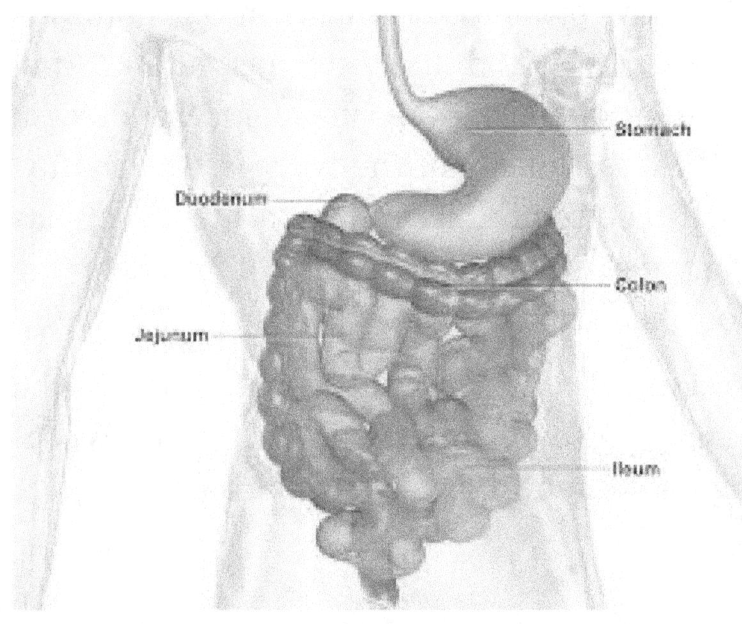

Mucus is an aqueous secretion produced by the cells of the mucous glands. It serves as a covering for the mucous membranes. Mucus is mainly composed of water, which is the mucin secretion.

It is an important element of the epithelial lining fluid, the airway surface liquid, which is the lining of the respiratory tract. Mucus helps to protect the lungs during breathing by trapping foreign particles and infectious agents like dust, allergens, virus, bacteria, etc.

The human body always tends to produce more mucus in order to protect and prevent the airway tissues from drying out. Thus, there is a continuous production of mucus in the respiratory system.

When foreign objects get trapped by the mucus, the mucus becomes thick and changes color most of the time. This thick mucus that is usually coughed out as sputum is known as phlegm.

Mucus also plays an important role in the digestive system. The layer formed by the mucus in the small intestine and colon helps to protect the intestinal epithelial cells from bacterial infections. It also serves as a lubricant for the movement of foods through the esophagus.

Interestingly, mucus is the body's natural lubricant in females which helps during sexual intercourse. It also helps to fight against infection in the reproductive system.

Mucus and the Health of the Body

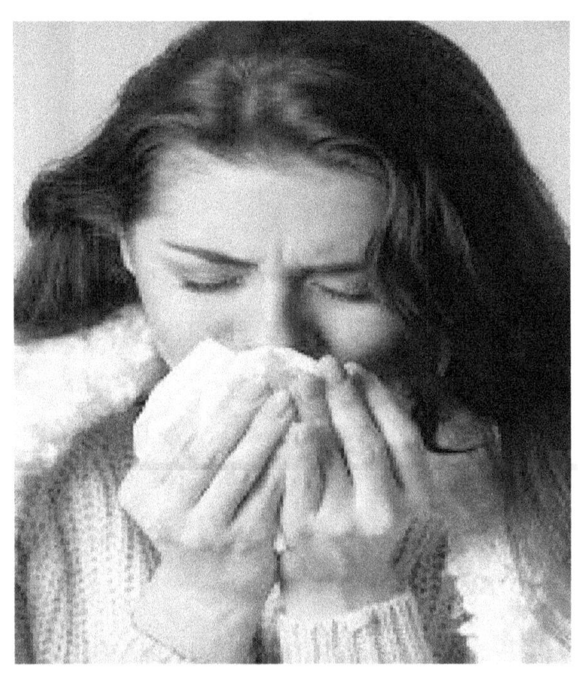

There is a continuous process of mucus production in the body, which helps to protect the body systems from infections and also provides necessary lubrication to the body.

Thus, the presence of mucus in our bodies is important. When mucus traps foreign and infectious bodies, it becomes phlegm. Phlegm and excess mucus in the body is not healthy. As the body produces up to a liter of mucus every day, it is vital to get rid of it to keep the body healthy.

Accumulation of mucus in the body is the major cause of illnesses as claimed by Dr. Sebi. So, excess mucus can be a red flag for an unhealthy state of the body.

Causes of Mucus Buildup in the Body

Just like in snails and other animals that secrete mucus, there are triggers for the production of mucus. In human beings, the major triggers are dryness and inflammation of the body. Some factors that may lead to dryness, inflammation, and other mucus secretion triggers are:

- Dry air
- Smoking
- Allergies
- Infections
- Acid reflux
- Asthma

- Low water/liquid consumption
- Medications etc.

These factors and more contribute to excess buildup of mucus in the body. The body naturally produces mucus to ensure that foreign objects (toxic and/or infectious) don't interact with the body cells. The more we have these foreign bodies, the more the body produces mucus.

When these objects get trapped by the mucus, the mucus becomes thick and builds up as phlegm.

Moreover, our body must stay lubricated for the swift movement of particles and cells in the body. Thus, dryness of the body makes the body produce more mucus, which is the liquid the body can produce naturally.

Chapter 2

ELECTRIC FOOD - ACID AND ALKALINE

Some foods and drinks change from acidic to alkaline once they are metabolized. This essentially makes them alkaline based, as once they are digested, they become alkaline. One of the most common foods in this category is citrus fruits, which contain ascorbic acid.

Citrus Fruits

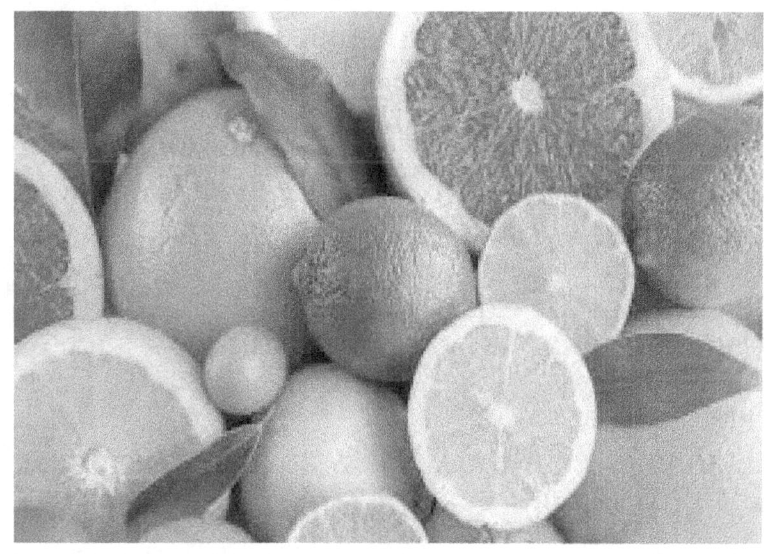

Citrus fruits may be often avoided as they are often considered acidic and sour to taste. Once they are fully digested, they effectively become alkaline in the body, with the results of increasing the pH balance to a more basic or alkaline environment. Fruits that fit into this category include lime, lemon, oranges, mandarins, tangerines, and grapefruit.

Tomatoes

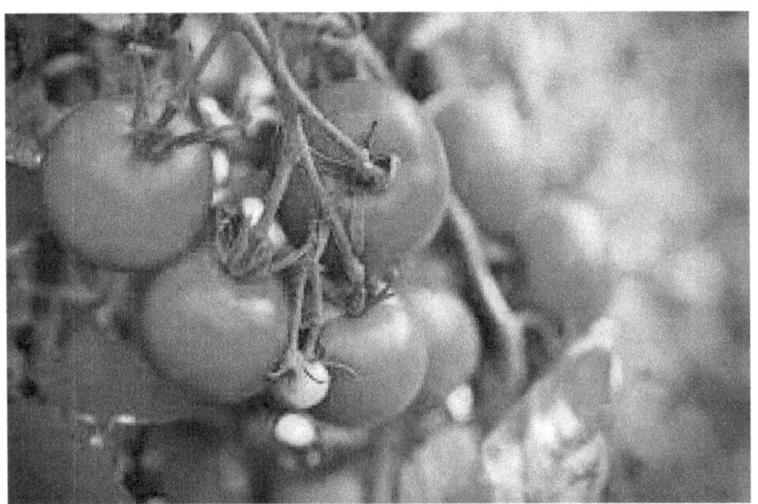

Tomatoes are another example of a fruit that becomes rich in alkaline once consumed. They are naturally acidic, and like citrus fruits, may be avoided due to their sour and sometimes strong taste. Tomatoes are best consumed in a raw state when they are digested quickly and increase the alkaline levels in the blood. When they are stewed, baked, or otherwise cooked, tomatoes increase in acidity, though are still very nutritious. If you enjoy tomatoes or cooked varieties are a regular part of your diet, incorporate both raw and cooked versions. For example, if you create pasta dishes, stew some tomatoes, and add some raw slices or cherry tomatoes as a topping to gain their benefits.

Kombucha Drinks

Kombucha is an acidic beverage that is comprised of fermented ingredients. It is typically created with a tea base (green or black tea), with added sugar for the fermentation process to form healthy bacterial cultures. There are many varieties of kombucha and recipes for flavoring and fermentation techniques. Kombucha drinks are growing in popularity in grocery stores and restaurants, though they were once considered a rare treat in upscale eateries and shops. They are available in many flavors and contain a longer shelf life than other fermented foods, such as yogurt, kimchi, and sauerkraut.

Why is kombucha beneficial for an alkaline diet? Although it is an acidic beverage, once metabolized, it becomes alkaline in the body. It is beneficial for gut health and aiding in the digestion process, which is due to the role of healthy bacteria, which also prevents infectious diseases and conditions, many of which originate in the gut. The healthy bacteria act as a barrier or protection in the stomach during the digestion process, which keeps acidic levels low to moderate. Kombucha is also high in antioxidants, which is a good defense against cancer, diabetes, and other conditions (for treatment and prevention), which is why this drink is beneficial as part of an alkaline diet.

Pineapples

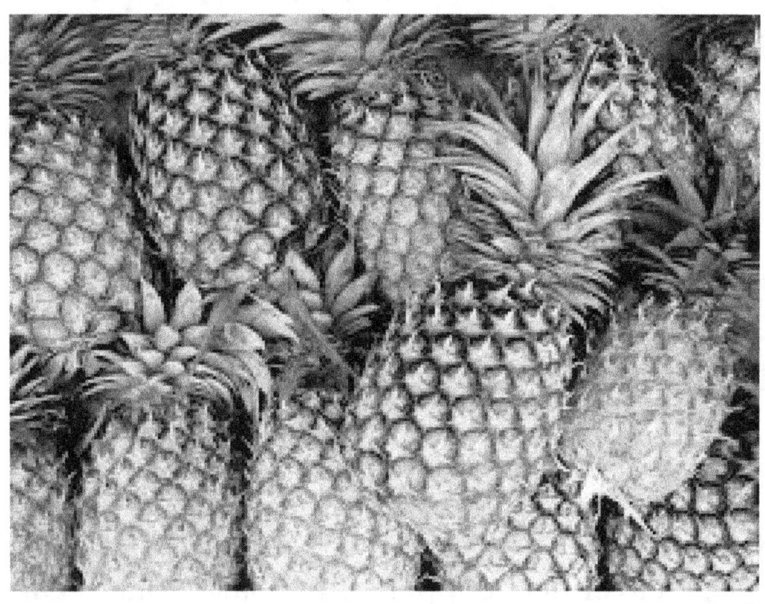

Many people will avoid pineapples because they can taste sour and cause irritation initially, though they are high in nutrients and alkalinize in the body once consumed. The benefits of pineapples include improving gut health, similarly, to fermented foods, such as yogurt and kombucha. Pineapples also reduce bloating and inflammation, which is caused by a lot of chronic and autoimmune conditions. Joint pain, arthritis, and other conditions that impact the bones and joints can be improved by the high amount of vitamin C and antioxidants in pineapples. Vitamin C improves the immunity function, which is beneficial for good health in general. If you exercise regularly and include weight or powerlifting as a part of your workout, eating pineapples and fruits high in vitamin C, fiber, and alkaline (once digested) can help your muscles recover quickly.

Apple Cider Vinegar

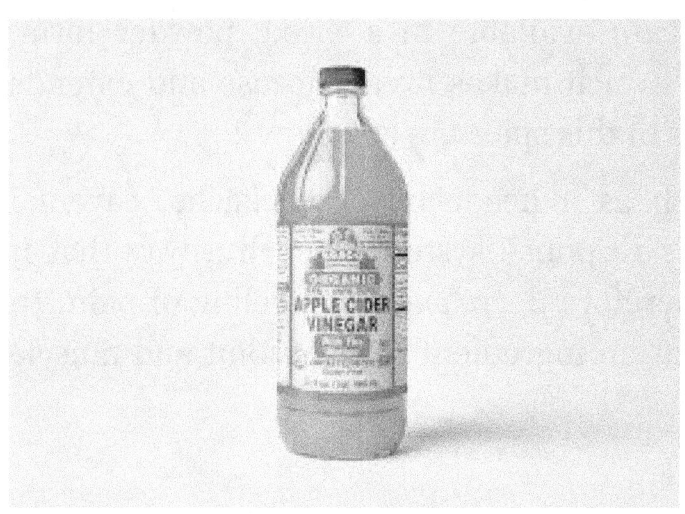

There are a lot of reported health benefits of adding apple cider vinegar to your diet, even in small amounts such as a tablespoon or two each day. This is made by mixing fermented apples with yeast and bacteria. Due to the acetic acid levels contained in it, many people avoid it altogether, as it has a pungent taste that is difficult to swallow. Diluting with water or lemon juice is one way to offset the strong taste, as well as adding to a balsamic dressing or another condiment. The benefits of apple cider vinegar work well with an alkaline diet for the following reasons:

Apple cider vinegar benefits insulin sensitivity and keeps blood sugar levels normal. While not conclusive, this effect may decrease the likelihood of developing type 2 diabetes.

Taken after a meal, it can help with the digestive process and curb overeating, which can promote weight loss and management.

It's best to consume with water or diluted with a similar drink such as tea or sparkling water to prevent the effects of the acetic acid on tooth enamel and the burning sensation on the mouth and throat if used regularly.

Hot Peppers (Including Cayenne Pepper)

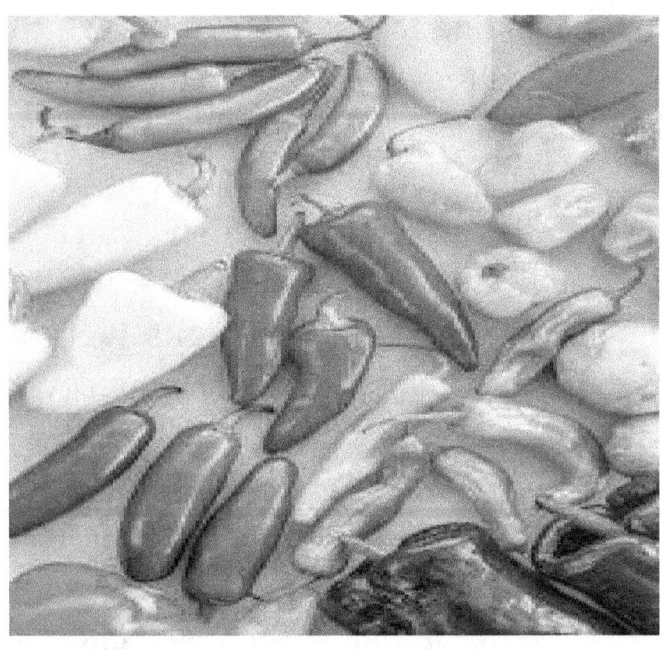

Peppers, the hot and spicy variety, and cayenne pepper, in particular, can provide a lot of health benefits. Most peppers are acidic naturally; though contain a lot of vitamin C and other nutrients that are good for your body. Cayenne pepper, specifically, becomes alkaline once it is ingested, which is a great reason to use as a seasoning in your meals, especially if you have a spicy palate. Most varieties of cayenne pepper are available in a dried, powder form, which makes it easy to use and extends the shelf life. The most important benefits of this spice are as follows:

When your body experiences pain, such as a headache or backache, cayenne provides a way of stimulating the body's response system in such a way that it diverts the sensation from the nerves, therefore decreasing the feeling of pain. In some natural remedies, cayenne is used as an ingredient to treat joint and muscle pain as a topical cream or oil.

There are some indications that cayenne pepper may aid with metabolism, which has a positive impact on weight loss. When your body produces heat, this increases the metabolism process. Cayenne pepper assists with this process, especially when enjoyed as part of a regular meal plan. While studies show that cayenne may not have consistent results in increasing metabolism over some time, it's important to note the initial benefit, as this can be a good way to start a weight loss plan.

Cayenne may suppress hunger, making you feel fuller faster and delaying the next meal or portion size. To make the most of this benefit, some people choose to take cayenne in a supplement form, such as capsules, which can usually be found in a natural health food store. If this is a supplement you want to include in your daily routine, consider finding the most natural, organic option available to ensure the maximum amount of benefits.

A lot of autoimmune conditions can be improved by changing diet, by alleviating symptoms to impact the underlying cause of the condition directly. One such condition is psoriasis, which is often treated with medications and topical creams. Capsaicin is an ingredient in cayenne, and as with creams for the treatment of joint and related pain relief, this ingredient is also used for psoriasis. Long-term benefits of reducing or possibly eliminating psoriasis by inhibiting the production of substance P in the body, which is primarily responsible for creating this condition.

Cayenne pepper is high in vitamin C and antioxidants, which can prevent and slow cancerous cell growth. Prostate, skin, and pancreatic cancers are among the types that can be prevented by cayenne pepper's nutritional ingredients.

The best benefit of cayenne pepper is how easy it is to add to most meals to enhance flavor. They are safe to eat and an excellent way to enjoy spicy food.

Chapter 3

ROLES AND FOOD PRINCIPLES

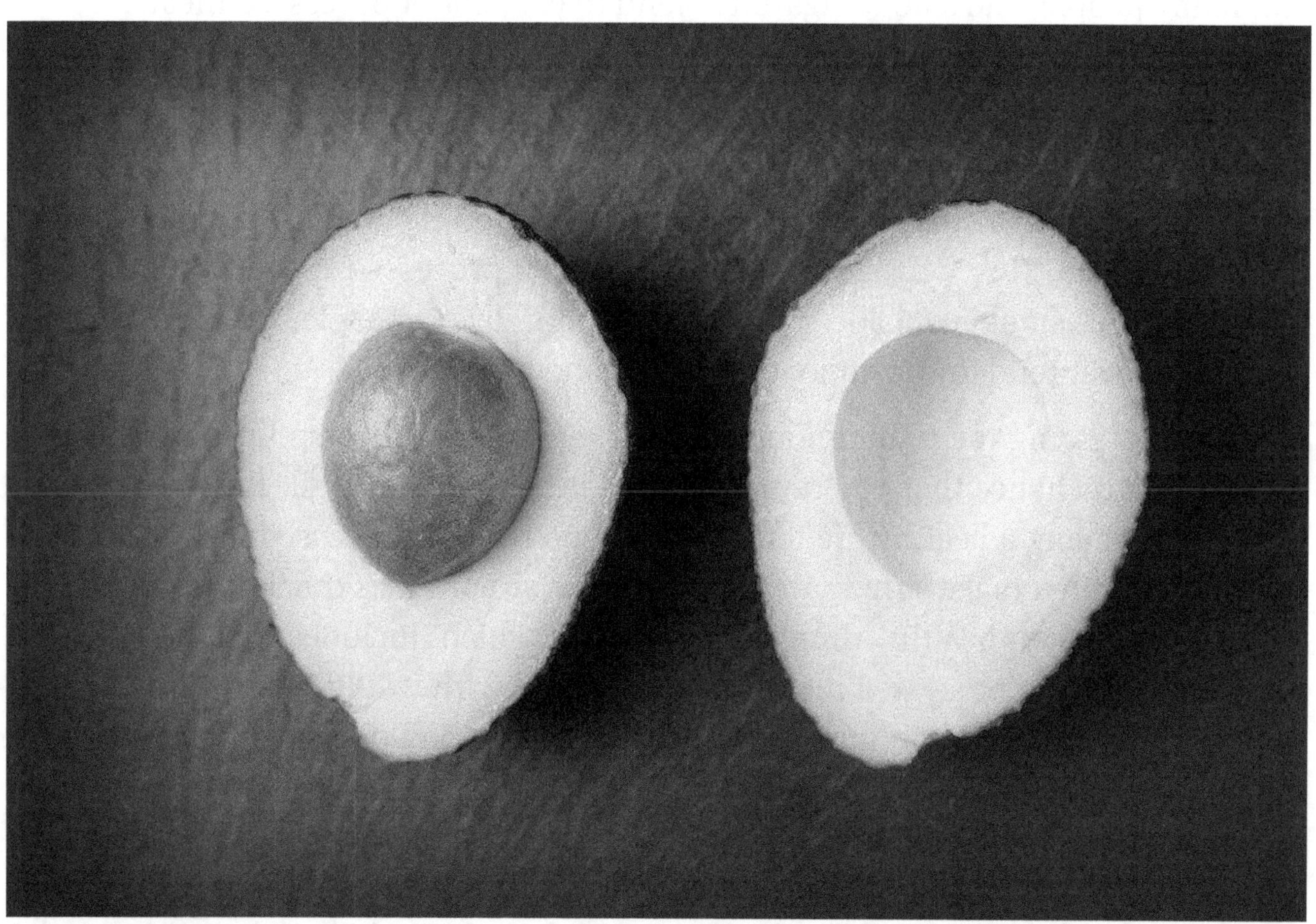

Even if you don't understand how most diets work, you know that processed meats are very bad for you when it comes to health and wellness. There have been many studies showing that processed meat can cause many diseases and illnesses. Moreover, they happen to be backed up with detailed studies to prove as such.

When following the alkaline diet, you are not allowed to eat any processed meat. It makes this diet one of the better diets when it comes to living a healthier life. Given all the benefits, you can now see how it can be an excellent idea for you to start following this diet.

Which is why they face more adversities when it comes to diseases in those specific areas; If you live in North America or a European country, then you will be facing a lot more of these diseases and problems. One of the most important things when it comes to eating processed meat is that it has been linked to an unhealthy lifestyle. Processed meat has been associated with being around people who are living an unhealthy life overall. Also, as you know, many people in the United States tend to live an unhealthy lifestyle and eat a ton of processed food. One example would be that many people who smoke cigarettes tend to eat a lot of processed meats.

Also, people who drink much alcohol will consume a lot of processed meat when they are intoxicated. This is a prevalent practice, which makes it a very unhealthy lifestyle decision. Ask yourself, when was the last time you consumed processed meat, there is a high chance that you were intoxicated the last time you consumed processed meat. Most of the time, you are eating processed meats when you are intoxicated or smoking a lot of cigarettes; moreover, people who eat a lot of processed meat tend to consume fewer fruits and vegetables.

If you're not eating the right amount of fiber and micronutrients in your diet, then there's a high chance that you're not living a healthy life overall. Basically, people who are not living a healthy life tend to consume a lot of processed meats. If you're one of them, then make sure that you rectify this situation as quickly as possible by cutting out the unhealthy things in your life which includes processed meat. Another thing that processed meat has been linked with would be chronic diseases. Eating processed meat can increase the risk of high blood pressure, heart diseases, cancer, and chronic obstructive pulmonary disease. There have been many studies showings, the people who eat this kind of meat tend to have a higher chance of attracting diseases stated above. There have also been studies done on an animal that has been consuming processed meat, and it showed that their cancer risk where bought higher when consuming processed meat as compared to when there were not.

The reason why is because processed meat contains harmful chemicals that may increase the risk of chronic diseases. There are numerous chemicals in processed meat; one of them is nitrite. This compound is one of the main reasons why your risk of cancer increases when consuming processed meat. This is the reason why the use of the compound is to preserve the red, pink color of the meat. It also helps to improve the taste of the meat and finally to get rid of any bacteria or growth in the long-term. Another reason why processed meat cannot be right for you is that it has been smoked. As we know, meat smoking is widespread when it comes to preservation.

It has often been salted and dried, to extend the shelf life of it. Once you get meat smoked in a burning wood and charcoal with dripping fat burns on a hot surface, it can cause many chemicals to form in the heat and hence making the meat very unhealthy. This is why it isn't a good idea to consume processed meats in the long-term, the way it has been made and processed makes it a terrible idea for you to consume it. There was one study done that showed when consuming processed meat every day equals smoking ten cigarettes a day in regard to the health effects you might face when consuming processed meat. This goes to show how bad processed meat can be for you. Another thing is that processed meat contains trans-fat. As you know, trans-fat is a human-made fat which has been causing many side effects on our health and wellness.

A decent amount of good fats in our diet is significant for optimal hormone production, etc. However, trans-fat can be very bad for us in the long term as it can cause many problems. One of the issues you might face when consuming trans-fat is the lowered amount of good cholesterol and the increase of bad cholesterol. Also, processed meat contains a lot of sodium, which can be very bad for us in the long-term. As you know, high amounts of sodium consumption can cause many illnesses and diseases. One of the significant things that it can cause is the risk of high blood pressure. High amounts of sodium have shown to increase blood pressure and inflammation increase, which is why it is not advisable for people to eat a lot of sodium when consuming processed meat. Processed meat can cause a lot of issues as we know by now, but one of the significant things that has been found in recent studies is that there is an increase in breast cancer.

There was one study that showed that when women consumed processed meat such as hot dogs, the risk of breast cancer went up 9%. This isn't high when you think about it, but it could still be avoided. Overall, the risk of type 2 diabetes will go up 19%, and the risk of heart disease while going up to 42% when consuming processed meat. These studies have been backed up by proper scientific studies done in a lab, which goes to show that processed meat cannot be good for health and overall well-being, which is one of the reasons why the alkaline diet does not allow you to eat meat in general, as a meat has been shown to increase the acidic levels in your body. The whole premise behind the alkaline diet is that you are not to consume foods that will raise your acidic level in your body when you have high acidic levels in your body, and there's a high chance for you to consume more bacteria. When there are more bacteria in your body, there's a high chance for you to attract more diseases and illnesses.

When it comes to attracting disease growing in your body, the bacteria like the acidic environment of your body, hence, when your body is sick, you will attract more of those diseases, and it will be more likely for you to grow them when your body is acidic. One of the most acidic things you can consume would be the use of processed meats. As you know, processed meats can cause many issues. If you're looking to follow the alkaline diet and then there's no chance in hell that you're going to be eating any processed meat. Even if you're someone looking to better your health, the first thing you need to do is cut out any processed meats that you think you're going to eat.

We can tell you what you should do and should not do, but as you can tell by the evidence that processed meat is not the answer when it comes to living a healthier life. More often than not, many of your consuming processed meat, and you don't even know it. Did you know that meats that are not organic and have been cut mechanically are also considered processed meats? These meats have been cut in a way that can cause many issues. Unfortunately, our system has made everything unhealthy when it comes to consuming food.

Chapter 4

WHAT TO EXPECT FROM THE DETOX

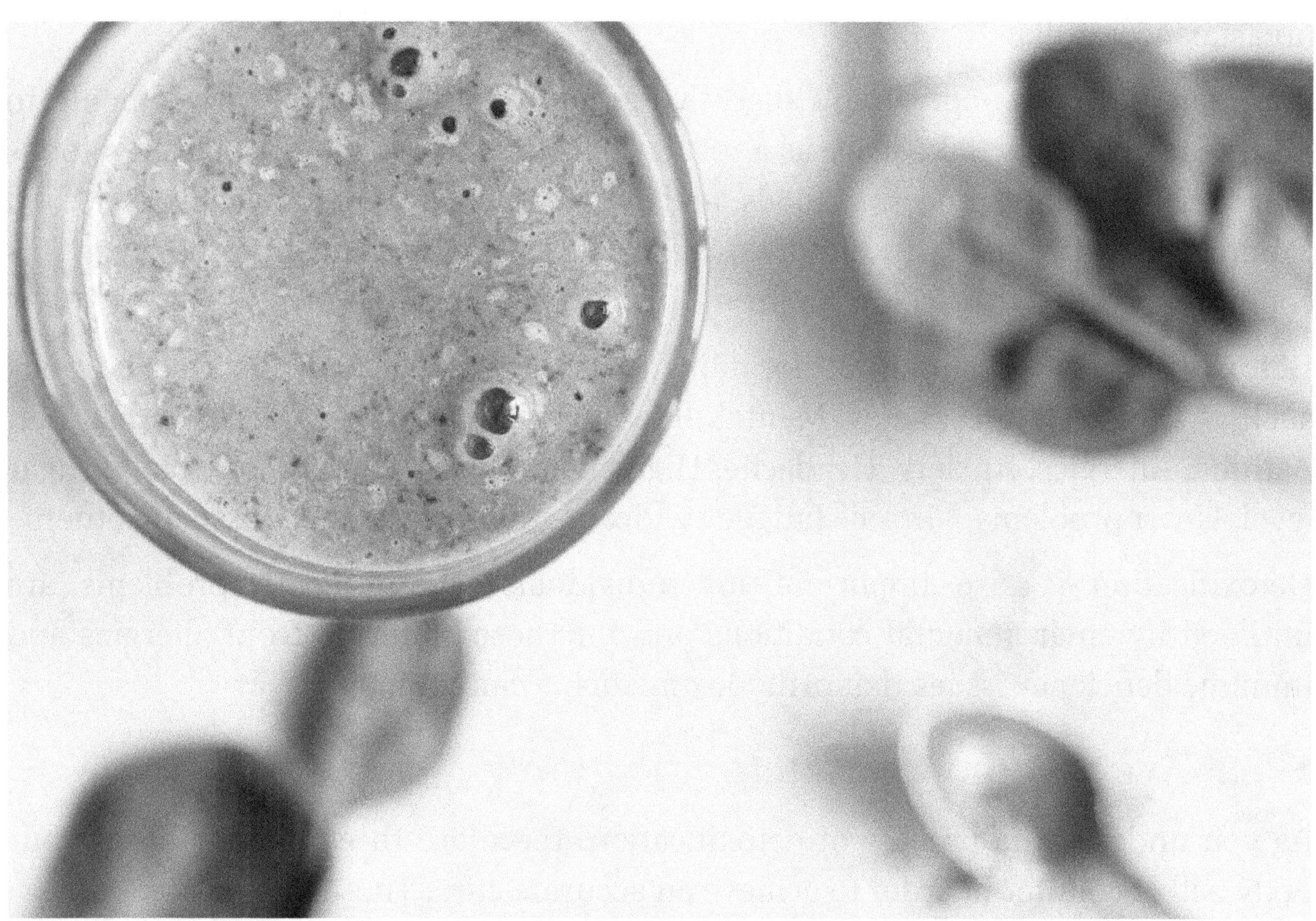

Detoxification is necessary when the body's natural detoxification organs become weak. This occurs as a result of prolonging the impact of stress, illness, poor health habit, improper diet, sedentary lifestyles, overconsumption of foods, exposure to environmental toxic substances, exposure to industrial by-products...and more.

A countless number of the toxic substances are opened to metabolic conversion or deactivation in the body and safely removed out of the body. But, when the body is loaded with environmental chemicals or when its detox organ (Liver) is not functioning well, toxins accumulate in fatty tissues and other body tissues.

Visible symptoms of this accumulation are chronic inflammation, constipation, fatigue, body odor, and overweight.

Some other dangerous effects are suppressed immune function, endocrine, and sexual dysfunction both in males and females, reduced male fertility, diabetes, increased risk for cardiovascular and liver disease.

Some chemicals found in skincare products (like Parabens) are associated with some hormones, accumulate in breast tissue, and excite the spread of human breast cancer cells.

For example, most individual's digestive systems that turn out to be unable to digest food properly; take place as a result of prolonging overconsumption of foods that are high in fats, processed foods, and low fiber foods. When this happens, food cannot move through the digestive tract and produce toxic by-products. This condition is called toxic colon syndrome or intestinal toxemia.

Detoxification is very important for individuals that have chronic health conditions such as Depression, Diabetes, Mental illness, Obesity, Cancer, Digestive disorder, Asthma, Allergies, Anxiety, Headache, High cholesterol, Arthritis, Low blood sugar level, Heart problems, Chronic fatigue syndrome, Fibromyalgia…and many others.

Detoxification is also important for individuals whose health problems are initiated by environmental conditions and for those suffering from allergies and immune deficiency issues that orthodox medicine cannot manage.

What Are the Phases of Detoxification?

As you undergo the process of detoxification, there are three major phases your body will encounter in order to achieve an accurate cure. These phases are:

Purification: in this process, you are expected to take in diets that are readily capable of detoxifying your body. This means that the diets you have to take in should be composed of detoxifying components. In this phase, you should endeavor to eat foods that are healthy and not unhealthy diets.

Restructuring/ reformation: at this phase, the body begins to adjust itself and encourages reformation. The whole system brings itself together to become healthy again.

Maintenance of good health: at this phase, the whole system interprets the information provided during the reformation phase and utilizes it to become perpetually healthy.

What Are the Benefits of Detoxification?

There are bundles of benefits you gain when you undergo the process of detoxification. These benefits are:

- It helps in weight loss and improves the well-being of the body.
- It helps in boosting the energy level.
- It helps in cleaning and strengthening the organs of detoxification and its passageways.
- It helps in boosting fertility in both men and women.
- It helps in improving mental functions.
- It helps in reducing fatigue.
- It helps in improving the appearance of the skin.
- It helps in the improvement of emotional wellbeing.
- It helps in improving memory.
- It helps in the enhancement of skin appearance.
- It helps in alleviating insomnia.
- It reduces the number of toxins in the body.
- It improves the circulatory system.
- It increases the body's immunity.
- It helps in improving optimal concentration.
- It helps in reducing stomach bloating.
- It provides strength for the nails and hair.
- It removes toxins from the liver.
- It helps in the improvement and strengthening of the digestive tract and system.
- It reduces the risk of diseases by improving the urinary system.

Chapter 5

7-Day Balanced Alkaline Detox Diet

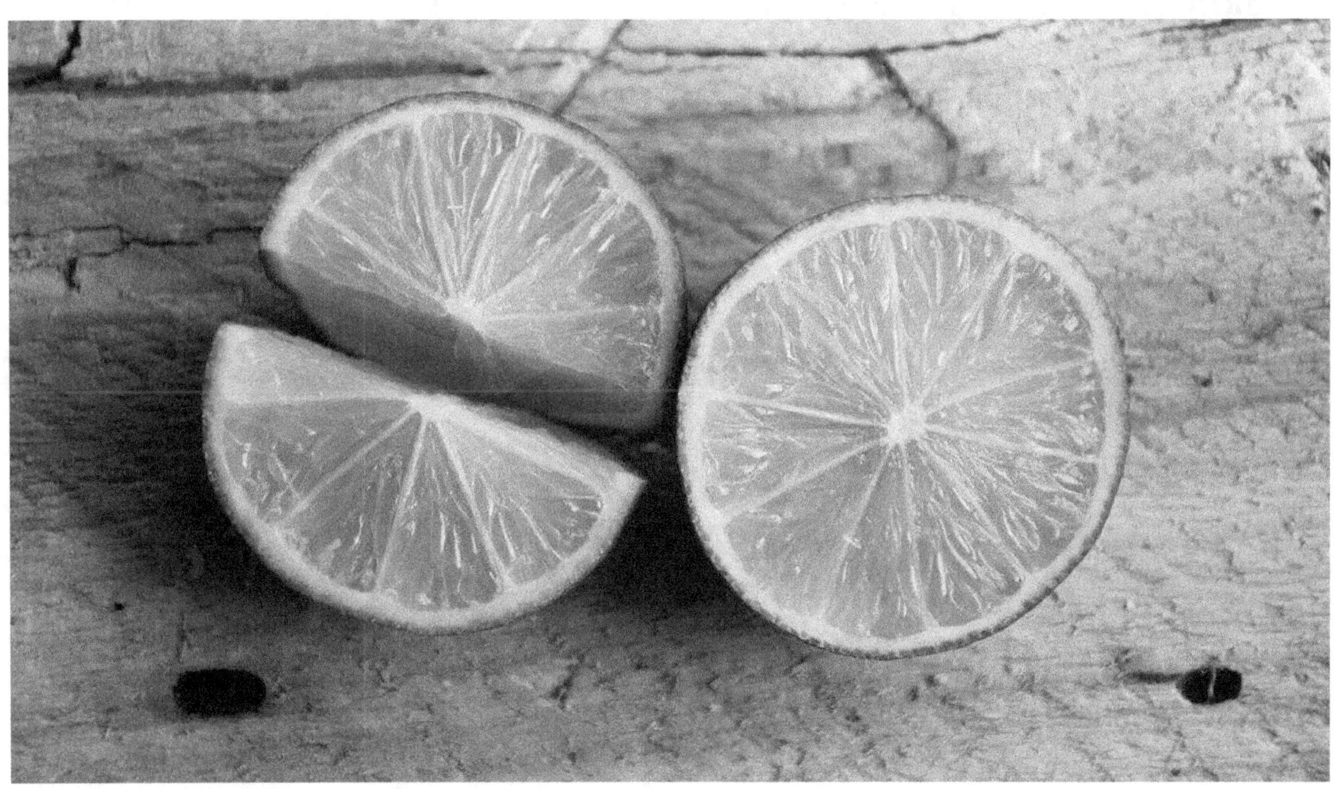

Detox Day One

Breakfast: Lime & Mint Summer Fruit Salad
Snack: Chives Chutney
Lunch: Crunchy Asparagus Spears
Dinner: Mini Turkey Meatloaves with Barbecue Sauce

Detox Day Two

Breakfast: Pumpkin Spice Quinoa
Snack: Cilantro Guacamole
Lunch: Quinoa Trail Mix Cups
Dinner: Mock Sangria

Detox Day Three

Breakfast: Jackfruit Vegetable Fry
Snack: Avocado Bites
Lunch: Oven Baked Sesame Fries
Dinner: Capriosa De Fresca

Detox Day Four

Breakfast: Banana Barley Porridge
Snack: Avocado and Radish Salsa
Lunch: Tofu & Bell Pepper Stew
Dinner: Adult Chocolate Milk with Spiced Rum

Detox Day Five

Breakfast: Zucchini Home Fries
Snack: Orange- Spiced Pumpkin Hummus
Lunch: Green Bean Casserole
Dinner: Warm Apple Delight

Detox Day Six

Breakfast: Millet Porridge
Snack: Cheesy Kale Chips
Lunch: Baked Beans
Dinner: Mock Sangria

Detox Day Seven

Breakfast: Turnip Bowl
Snack: Mini Nacho Pizzas
Lunch: Cinnamon Apple Chips with Dip
Dinner: Mixed Berry Crisp

Chapter 6

BREAKFAST RECIPES

1. Vegetable Pancakes

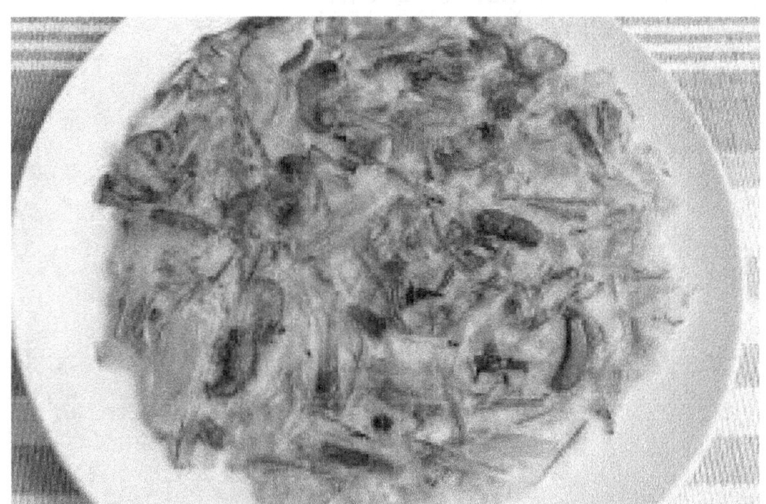

Preparation Time: 5 minutes

Cooking Time: 5 minutes

Serving: 2

Ingredients:

- ½ white onion, grated
- 1 yellow squash, roughly chopped
- 1 zucchini, peeled and chopped
- 1 zucchini, roughly chopped
- ½ teaspoon onion powder

- ¼ cup filtered water, as needed
- 1 teaspoon salt
- ¼ cup coconut flour
- 4 scallions

Directions:

1. Add the yellow squash, zucchini, zucchini, scallions, coconut flour, onion, salt, and onion powder in a food processor. Pulse until blended.
2. Add the water to the mixture to make moist but not runny. The batter will be thick.
3. Spray Pan with cooking spray and heat over medium-high heat.
4. Using an ice-cream scoop to drop batter into the pan. Use a fork to spread your mixture evenly over the pan, pressing down on the pancakes. Brown on both sides of pancakes, cooking for about 5 minutes total.
5. Serve hot and enjoy!

Nutrition: calories 254 fat 12.1 carbs 33.4 protein 6.3

2. Turnip Bowl

Preparation Time: 5 minutes

Cooking Time: 10 minutes

Serving: 2

Ingredients:

- 2 turnips, peeled and cubed
- 1 tablespoon coconut oil
- 1 red bell pepper, seeded and chopped
- 1 sweet onion, chopped
- ¼ cup mushrooms, sliced
- 4 cups kale
- 2 chive stalks, chopped
- 1 teaspoon onion powder
- 1 teaspoon onion powder
- ½ teaspoon sea salt

- ½ teaspoon bouquet garn herb blended, or other dried herbs like sage or rosemary

Directions:

1. In a bowl, combine the turnips, red bell pepper, mushrooms, kale, chives, onion, oil, onion powder, and onion powder.
2. Heat a non-stick cooking pan over medium heat, and cook the vegetables, stirring often for about 10 minutes, or until tender.
3. Serve and Enjoy!

Nutrition: calories 190, fat 2, carbs 18, protein 11

3. Millet Porridge

Preparation Time: 10 minutes

Cooking Time: 20 minutes

Serving: 2

Ingredients:

- Pinch of sea salt
- 1 tablespoon coconuts, chopped finely
- ½ cup unsweetened coconut milk
- ½ cup millet, rinsed and drained
- 1½ cups water
- 3 drops liquid stevia

Directions:

1. Sauté millet in a non-stick skillet for 3 minutes. Stir in salt and water. Let it boil then reduce the heat.
2. Cook for 15 minutes then stirs in remaining ingredients. Cook for another 4 minutes.
3. Serve with chopped nuts on top.

Nutrition: calories 219, fat 5, carbs 38, protein 6

4. Jackfruit Vegetable Fry

Preparation Time: 5 minutes

Cooking Time: 5 minutes

Serving: 6

Ingredients:

- 2 small onions, finely chopped
- 2 cups cherry tomatoes, finely chopped
- 1/8 teaspoon ground turmeric
- 1 tablespoon olive oil
- 2 red bell peppers, seeded and chopped
- 3 cups firm jackfruit, seeded and chopped
- 1/8 teaspoon cayenne pepper
- 2 tablespoons fresh basil leaves, chopped
- Salt, to taste

Directions:

1. Sauté onions and bell peppers in a greased skillet for 5 minutes. Stir in tomatoes and cook for 2 minutes.
2. Add turmeric, salt, cayenne pepper, and jackfruit. Cook for 8 minutes.
3. Garnish with basil leaves. Serve warm.

Nutrition: calories 237, fat 2, carbs 28, protein 7

5. Zucchini Pancakes

Preparation Time: 15 minutes

Cooking Time: 8 minutes

Serving: 8

Ingredients:

- 12 tablespoons water
- 6 large zucchinis, grated
- Sea salt, to taste
- 4 tablespoons ground Flax Seeds

- 2 teaspoons olive oil
- 2 jalapeño peppers, finely chopped
- ½ cup scallions, finely chopped

Directions:

1. Mix together water and flax seeds in a bowl and keep aside.
2. Heat oil in a large non-stick skillet on medium heat and add zucchini, salt, and black pepper.
3. Cook for about 3 minutes and transfer the zucchini into a large bowl. Stir in scallions and flaxseed mixture and thoroughly mix.
4. Preheat a griddle and grease it lightly with cooking spray. Pour about ¼ of the zucchini mixture into a preheated griddle and cook for about 3 minutes.
5. Flip the side carefully and cook for about 2 more minutes. Repeat with the remaining mixture in batches and serve.

Nutrition: calories 90, fat 3, carbs 22, protein 11

6. Squash Hash

Preparation Time: 2 minutes

Cooking Time: 10 minutes

Serving: 2

Ingredients:

- 1 teaspoon onion powder
- ½ cup onion, finely chopped
- 2 cups spaghetti squash
- ½ teaspoon sea salt

Directions:

1. Squeeze any extra moisture from spaghetti squash using paper towels. Place the squash into a bowl, then add the onion powder, onion, and salt. Stir to combine.
2. Spray a non-stick cooking skillet with cooking spray and place it over medium heat.

3. Add the spaghetti squash to the pan. Cook the squash for 5 minutes, untouched. Using a spatula, flip the hash browns. Cook for an additional 5 minutes or until the desired crispness is reached. Serve and Enjoy!

Nutrition: calories 212, fat 6, carbs 10, protein 10

7. Hemp Seed Porridge

Preparation Time: 5 minutes

Cooking Time: 5 minutes

Serving: 6

Ingredients:

- Hemp seed
- Stevia
- Coconut milk

Directions:

1. Combine the rice and coconut milk in a saucepan over medium heat for 5 minutes. Make sure to stir constantly.
2. Remove the pan from the heat and stir in the Stevia.
3. Divide among 6 bowls.
4. Serve and Enjoy!

Nutrition: calories 219, fat 2, carbs 18, protein 7

8. Veggie Medley

Preparation Time: 5 minutes

Cooking Time: 10 minutes

Serving:

Ingredients:

- 1 bell pepper, any color, seeded and sliced
- Juice of ½ a lime
- 2 tablespoons fresh cilantro
- ½ teaspoon cumin

- 1 teaspoon sea salt
- 1 jalapeno, chopped
- ½ cup zucchini, sliced
- 1 cup cherry tomatoes, halved
- ½ cup mushrooms, sliced
- 1 cup broccoli florets, cooked
- 1 sweet onion, chopped

Directions:

1. Spray a non-stick pan with cooking spray and place it over medium heat.
2. Add the onion, broccoli, bell pepper, tomatoes, zucchini, mushrooms, and jalapeno. Cook for 7 minutes, or until the desired doneness is reached. Stir occasionally.
3. Stir in the cumin, cilantro, and salt. Cook for 3 minutes while stirring.
4. Remove pan from heat, then add the lime juice.
5. Divide between serving plates, serve, and enjoy!

Nutrition: calories 89, fat 2, carbs 17, protein 5

9. Pumpkin Spice Quinoa

Preparation Time: 10 minutes

Cooking Time: 0 min

Serving: 2

Ingredients:

- 1 cup cooked quinoa
- 1 cup unsweetened coconut milk
- 1 large banana, mashed
- 1/4 cup pumpkin puree
- 1 teaspoon pumpkin spice
- 2 teaspoon chia seeds

Directions:

1. Mix all the ingredients in a container.
2. Seal the lid and shake well to mix.

3. Refrigerate overnight.
4. Serve.

Nutrition: calories 213, fat 6, carbs 18, protein 7

10. Zucchini Home Fries

Preparation Time: 5 minutes

Cooking Time: 20 minutes

Serving: 2

Ingredients:

- 4 medium zucchinis
- 1 teaspoon onion powder
- 1 teaspoon sea salt
- 1 red bell pepper, seeded, diced
- ½ sweet white onion, chopped
- ¼ cup vegetable broth
- ½ cup mushrooms, sliced

Directions:

1. In a medium-sized microwave-safe bowl, microwave the 4 zucchinis for about 4 minutes or until soft. Allow zucchinis to cool.
2. Add the broth into a large non-stick pan over medium heat, add the red bell pepper and onion. Sauté your vegetables for 5 minutes.
3. While the vegetables are cooking, slice your zucchinis into quarters.
4. Add the mushrooms, onion powder, salt, and zucchinis to the pan. Cook your mixture for about 10 minutes or until the zucchinis are crisp.
5. Serve and Enjoy!

Nutrition: calories 332, fat 1, carbs 34, protein 9

11. Figs & Ginger Fruit Compote

Preparation Time: 10 minutes

Cooking Time: 10 minutes

Serving: 4

Ingredients:

- 1 apple, peeled, cored, and diced
- 2 tangerines, peeled and sectioned
- ½ cup plums, dried and halved
- ½ cup figs, stemmed and quartered
- 1 packet Stevia
- ½ teaspoon cloves
- ½ teaspoon cinnamon
- 1 teaspoon ginger, fresh and grated
- 1 vanilla bean, split lengthwise, deseeded
- ¼ cup dark cherries
- 1 cup of filtered water

Directions:

1. In a saucepan, mix all of the ingredients.
2. Bring to a simmer over medium heat and cook for 10 minutes, stirring occasionally or until the fruit is tender.
3. Remove from the heat source, then let stand for 30 minutes.
4. Serve warm and Enjoy!

Nutrition: calories 102, fat 1, carbs 26, protein 1

12. Lime & Mint Summer Fruit Salad

Preparation Time: 10 minutes

Cooking Time: 0 minutes

Serving: 4

Ingredients:

- ¼ cup apple, peeled and diced
- ¼ cup grapes
- 2 tablespoons mint, fresh and chopped
- 2 tablespoons Seville orange juice, freshly squeezed
- ¼ cup strawberries
- ¼ cup peaches, peeled and diced

- ¼ cup tangerine slices
- ¼ cup cantaloupe, small bite-size pieces
- ¼ cup honeydew melon, small bite-size pieces
- ¼ cup watermelon, small bite-size pieces

Directions:

1. In a mixing bowl, combine all of the fruit.
2. Add the Seville orange juice, mint, and mix well.
3. Serve chilled and enjoy!

Nutrition: calories 150, fat 1, carbs 7, protein 2

13. Banana Barley Porridge

Preparation Time: 5 minutes

Cooking Time: 30 minutes

Serving: 2

Ingredients:

- 1 cup unsweetened coconut milk, divided
- 1 small banana, peeled and sliced
- ½ cup barley
- 3 drops liquid stevia
- ¼ cup coconuts, chopped

Directions:

1. Mix barley with half coconut milk and stevia in a bowl and mix well. Cover and refrigerate for about 6 hours.
2. Mix the barley mixture with coconut milk in a saucepan. Cook for 5 minutes on medium heat.
3. Top with chopped coconuts and banana slices. Serve.

Nutrition: calories 420, fat 3, carbs 28, protein 7

14. Zucchini Muffins

Preparation Time: 10 minutes

Cooking Time: 25 minutes

Serving: 16

Ingredients:

- 1 tablespoon ground flaxseed
- 3 tablespoons water
- ¼ cup walnut butter
- 3 small-medium over-ripe bananas
- 2 small zucchinis, grated
- ½ cup coconut milk
- 1 teaspoon vanilla extract
- 2 cups coconut flour
- 1 tablespoon baking powder
- 1 teaspoon cinnamon
- ¼ teaspoon sea salt
- Optional add-ins:
- ¼ cup chocolate chips and/or walnuts

Directions:

1. Set your oven to 375 degrees F. Grease a muffin tray with cooking spray. Mix flaxseed with water in a bowl.
2. Mash bananas in a glass bowl and stir in all the remaining ingredients. Mix well and divide the mixture into the muffin tray.
3. Bake for 25 minutes. Serve.

Nutrition: calories 170, fat 4, carbs 13, protein 1

15. Millet Porridge

Preparation Time: 10 minutes

Cooking Time: 20 minutes

Serving: 2

Ingredients:

- Pinch of sea salt
- 1 tablespoon coconuts, chopped finely
- ½ cup unsweetened coconut milk
- ½ cup millet, rinsed and drained
- 1½ cups water
- 3 drops liquid stevia

Directions:

1. Sauté millet in a non-stick skillet for 3 minutes. Stir in salt and water. Let it boil then reduce the heat.
2. Cook for 15 minutes then stirs in remaining ingredients. Cook for another 4 minutes.
3. Serve with chopped nuts on top.

Nutrition: calories 219, fat 2, carbs 8, protein 6

16. Jackfruit Vegetable Fry

Preparation Time: 5 minutes

Cooking Time: 5 minutes

Serving: 6

Ingredients:

- 2 small onions, finely chopped
- 2 cups cherry tomatoes, finely chopped
- 1/8 teaspoon ground turmeric
- 1 tablespoon olive oil
- 2 red bell peppers, seeded and chopped
- 3 cups firm jackfruit, seeded and chopped
- 1/8 teaspoon cayenne pepper
- 2 tablespoons fresh basil leaves, chopped
- Salt, to taste

Directions:

1. Sauté onions and bell peppers in a greased skillet for 5 minutes. Stir in tomatoes and cook for 2 minutes.
2. Add turmeric, salt, cayenne pepper, and jackfruit. Cook for 8 minutes.
3. Garnish with basil leaves. Serve warm.

Nutrition: calories 236, fat 2, carbs 10, protein 7

17. Zucchini Pancakes

Preparation Time: 15 minutes

Cooking Time: 8 minutes

Serving: *8*

Ingredients:

- 12 tablespoons water
- 6 large zucchinis, grated
- Sea salt, to taste
- 4 tablespoons ground Flax Seeds
- 2 teaspoons olive oil
- 2 jalapeño peppers, finely chopped
- ½ cup scallions, finely chopped

Directions:

1. Mix together water and flax seeds in a bowl and keep aside.
2. Heat oil in a large non-stick skillet on medium heat and add zucchini, salt, and black pepper.
3. Cook for about 3 minutes and transfer the zucchini into a large bowl. Stir in scallions and flaxseed mixture and thoroughly mix.
4. Preheat a griddle and grease it lightly with cooking spray. Pour about ¼ of the zucchini mixture into a preheated griddle and cook for about 3 minutes.
5. Flip the side carefully and cook for about 2 more minutes. Repeat with the remaining mixture in batches and serve.

Nutrition: calories 132, fat 3, carbs 9, protein 4

18. Squash Hash

Preparation Time: 2 minutes

Cooking Time: 10 minutes

Serving: 2

Ingredients:

- 1 teaspoon onion powder
- ½ cup onion, finely chopped
- 2 cups spaghetti squash
- ½ teaspoon sea salt

Directions:

1. Squeeze any extra moisture from spaghetti squash using paper towels. Place the squash into a bowl, then add the onion powder, onion, and salt. Stir to combine.
2. Spray a non-stick cooking skillet with cooking spray and place it over medium heat.
3. Add the spaghetti squash to the pan. Cook the squash for 5 minutes, untouched. Using a spatula, flip the hash browns. Cook for an additional 5 minutes or until the desired crispness is reached. Serve and Enjoy!

Nutrition: calories 180, fat 2, carbs 8, protein 1

19. Veggie Medley

Preparation Time: 5 minutes

Cooking Time: 10 minutes

Serving: 2

Ingredients:

- 1 bell pepper, any color, seeded and sliced
- Juice of ½ a lime
- 2 tablespoons fresh cilantro
- ½ teaspoon cumin
- 1 teaspoon sea salt

- 1 jalapeno, chopped
- ½ cup zucchini, sliced
- 1 cup cherry tomatoes, halved
- ½ cup mushrooms, sliced
- 1 cup broccoli florets, cooked
- 1 sweet onion, chopped

Directions:

1. Spray a non-stick pan with cooking spray and place it over medium heat.
2. Add the onion, broccoli, bell pepper, tomatoes, zucchini, mushrooms, and jalapeno. Cook for 7 minutes, or until the desired doneness is reached. Stir occasionally.
3. Stir in the cumin, cilantro, and salt. Cook for 3 minutes while stirring.
4. Remove pan from heat, then add the lime juice.
5. Divide between serving plates, serve, and enjoy!

Nutrition: calories 90, fat 2, carbs 16, protein 4

20. Pumpkin Spice Quinoa

Preparation Time: 10 minutes

Cooking Time: 0 min

Serving: 2

Ingredients:

- 1 cup cooked quinoa
- 1 cup unsweetened coconut milk
- 1 large banana, mashed
- 1/4 cup pumpkin puree
- 1 teaspoon pumpkin spice
- 2 teaspoon chia seeds

Directions:

1. Mix all the ingredients in a container.
2. Seal the lid and shake well to mix.
3. Refrigerate overnight.

4. Serve.

Nutrition: calories 216, fat 2, carbs 18, protein 9

21. Zucchini Home Fries

Preparation Time: 5 minutes

Cooking Time: 20 minutes

Serving: 2

Ingredients:

- 4 medium zucchinis
- 1 teaspoon onion powder
- 1 teaspoon sea salt
- 1 red bell pepper, seeded, diced
- ½ sweet white onion, chopped
- ¼ cup vegetable broth
- ½ cup mushrooms, sliced

Directions:

1. In a medium-sized microwave-safe bowl, microwave the 4 zucchinis for about 4 minutes or until soft. Allow zucchinis to cool.
2. Add the broth into a large non-stick pan over medium heat, add the red bell pepper and onion. Sauté your vegetables for 5 minutes.
3. While the vegetables are cooking, slice your zucchinis into quarters.
4. Add the mushrooms, onion powder, salt, and zucchinis to the pan. Cook your mixture for about 10 minutes or until the zucchinis are crisp.
5. Serve and Enjoy!

Nutrition: calories 321, fat 2, carbs 28, protein 11

22. Figs & Ginger Fruit Compote

Preparation Time: 10 minutes

Cooking Time: 10 minutes

Serving: 4

Ingredients:

- 1 apple, peeled, cored, and diced
- 2 tangerines, peeled and sectioned
- ½ cup plums, dried and halved
- ½ cup figs, stemmed and quartered
- 1 packet stevia
- ½ teaspoon cloves
- ½ teaspoon cinnamon
- 1 teaspoon ginger, fresh and grated
- 1 vanilla bean, split lengthwise, deseeded
- ¼ cup dark cherries
- 1 cup of filtered water

Directions:

1. In a saucepan, mix all of the ingredients.
2. Bring to a simmer over medium heat and cook for 10 minutes, stirring occasionally or until the fruit is tender.
3. Remove from the heat source, then let stand for 30 minutes.
4. Serve warm and Enjoy!

Nutrition: calories 130, fat 1, carbs 26, protein 1

23. Lime & Mint Summer Fruit Salad

Preparation Time: 10 minutes

Cooking Time: 0 minutes

Serving: 4

Ingredients:

- ¼ cup apple, peeled and diced
- ¼ cup grapes
- 2 tablespoons mint, fresh and chopped
- 2 tablespoons Seville orange juice, freshly squeezed
- ¼ cup strawberries
- ¼ cup peaches, peeled and diced

- ¼ cup tangerine slices
- ¼ cup cantaloupe, small bite-size pieces
- ¼ cup honeydew melon, small bite-size pieces
- ¼ cup watermelon, small bite-size pieces

Directions:

1. In a mixing bowl, combine all of the fruit.
2. Add the Seville orange juice, mint, and mix well.
3. Serve chilled and enjoy!

Nutrition: calories 86, fat 0, carbs 7, protein 1

24. Dr. Sebi Granola

Preparation Time: 2 minutes

Cooking Time: 15 minutes

Serving: 4

Ingredients:

- 1 cup slivered coconuts
- 1 cup flaked unsweetened coconut
- ½ cup raisins
- ½ cup flaxseed
- ½ teaspoon nutmeg
- ½ teaspoon cinnamon
- ¼ teaspoon ginger
- ¼ teaspoon sea salt
- ½ cup unsweetened dried pineapple pieces
- ¼ cup coconut oil

Directions:

1. Preheat your oven to 350° Fahrenheit.
2. In a bowl, combine the coconut, flaxseed, coconuts, raisins, ginger, cinnamon, nutmeg, vanilla bean seeds, salt, and coconut oil. Mix until well combined.

3. Spread the mix on a baking sheet and bake for 15 minutes, occasionally stirring, until golden brown.
4. Remove from your oven and cool, without stirring.
5. Once cooled, stir in the pineapple pieces.
6. Store in an airtight container.

Nutrition: calories 219, fat 1, carbs 18, protein 1

25. Vegetable Pancakes

Preparation Time: 5 minutes

Cooking Time: 5 minutes

Serving: 2

Ingredients:

- ½ white onion, grated
- 1 yellow squash, roughly chopped
- 1 zucchini, peeled and chopped
- 1 zucchini, roughly chopped
- ½ teaspoon onion powder
- ¼ cup filtered water, as needed
- 1 teaspoon salt
- ¼ cup coconut flour
- 4 scallions

Directions:

1. Add the yellow squash, zucchini, zucchini, scallions, coconut flour, onion, salt, and onion powder in a food processor. Pulse until blended.
2. Add the water to the mixture to make moist but not runny. The batter will be thick.
3. Spray Pan with cooking spray and heat over medium-high heat.
4. Using an ice-cream scoop to drop batter into the pan. Use a fork to spread your mixture evenly over the pan, pressing down on the pancakes. Brown on both sides of pancakes, cooking for about 5 minutes total.
5. Serve hot and Enjoy!

Nutrition: calories 140, fat 1, carbs 8, protein 1

26. Turnip Bowl

Preparation Time: 5 minutes

Cooking Time: 10 minutes

Serving: 2

Ingredients:

- 2 turnips, peeled and cubed
- 1 tablespoon coconut oil
- 1 red bell pepper, seeded and chopped
- 1 sweet onion, chopped
- ¼ cup mushrooms, sliced
- 4 cups kale
- 2 chive stalks, chopped
- 1 teaspoon onion powder
- 1 teaspoon onion powder
- ½ teaspoon sea salt
- ½ teaspoon Bouquet Garn herb blended, or other dried herbs like sage or rosemary

Directions:

1. In a bowl, combine the turnips, red bell pepper, mushrooms, kale, chives, onion, oil, onion powder, and onion powder.
2. Heat a non-stick cooking pan over medium heat, and cook the vegetables, stirring often for about 10 minutes, or until tender.
3. Serve and Enjoy!

Nutrition: calories 211, fat 1, carbs 9, protein 1

Chapter 7

SMOOTHIES

27. Pineapple, Banana & Spinach Smoothie

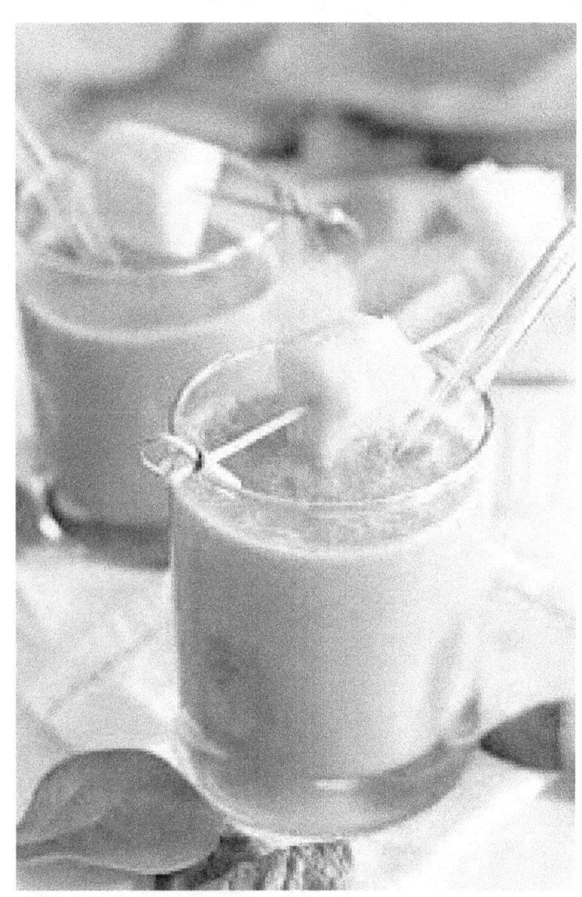

Preparation Time: 10 Minutes

Cooking time: 0 minute

Servings: 1

Ingredients:

- ½ cup almond milk
- ¼ cup soy yogurt
- 1 cup spinach
- 1 cup banana
- 1 cup pineapple chunks
- 1 tbsp. chia seeds

Directions:

1. Add all the ingredients to a blender.
2. Blend until smooth.
3. Chill in the refrigerator before serving.

Nutrition: calories 153, fat 1, carbs 8, protein 1

28. Kale & Avocado Smoothie

Preparation Time: 10 Minutes

Cooking time: 0 minute

Servings: 1

Ingredients:

- 1 ripe banana
- 1 cup kale
- 1 cup almond milk
- ¼ avocado
- 1 tbsp. chia seeds
- 2 tsp. honey
- 1 cup ice cubes

Direction:

1. Blend all the ingredients until smooth.

Nutrition: calories 133, fat 1, carbs 9, protein 1

29. Coconut & Strawberry Smoothie

Preparation Time: 10 Minutes

Cooking Time: 0 minutes

Serves: 1

Ingredients:

- 1 Cup Strawberries, Frozen & Thawed Slightly
- 1 Ripe Banana, Sliced & Frozen
- ½ Cup Coconut Milk, Light
- ½ Cup Vegan Yogurt
- 1 Tablespoon Chia Seeds
- 1 Teaspoon Lime juice, Fresh
- 4 Ice Cubes

Directions:

1. Blend everything together until smooth and serve immediately.

Nutrition: calories 210, fat 2, carbs 7, protein 9

30. Pumpkin Chia Smoothie

Preparation Time: 5 Minutes

Cooking Time: 0 minutes

Servings: 1

Ingredients:

- 3 Tablespoons Pumpkin Puree
- 1 Tablespoon MCT Oil
- ¾ Cup Coconut Milk, Full Fat
- ½ Avocado, Fresh
- 1 Teaspoon Vanilla, Pure
- ½ Teaspoon Pumpkin Pie Spice

Directions:

1. Combine all ingredients together until blended.

Nutrition: calories 188, fat 1, carbs 9, protein 1

31. Cantaloupe Smoothie Bowl

Preparation Time: 5 Minutes

Cooking Time: 0 minutes

Servings: 2

Ingredients:

- ¾ cup carrot juice
- 4 cups cantaloupe, frozen & cubed
- Melon balls or berries to serve
- Pinch sea salt

Directions:

1. Blend everything together until smooth.

Nutrition: calories 105, fat 1, carbs 3, protein 9

32. Berry & Cauliflower Smoothie

Preparation Time: 10 Minutes

Cooking Time: 0 minutes

Servings: 2

Ingredients:

- 1 Cup Riced Cauliflower, Frozen
- 1 Cup Banana, Sliced & Frozen
- ½ Cup Mixed Berries, Frozen
- 2 Cups Almond Milk, Unsweetened
- 2 Teaspoons Maple syrup, Pure & Optional

Directions:

1. Blend until mixed well.

Nutrition: calories 122, fat 1, carbs 4, protein 10

33. Green Mango Smoothie

Preparation Time: 5 Minutes

Cooking Time: 0 minutes

Servings: 1

Ingredients:

- 2 Cups Spinach
- 1-2 Cups Coconut Water
- 2 Mangos, Ripe, Peeled & Diced

Directions:

1. Blend everything together until smooth.

Nutrition: calories 120, fat 1, carbs 5, protein 8

34. Chia Seed Smoothie

Preparation Time: 5 Minutes

Cooking Time: 0 minutes

Servings: 3

Ingredients:

- ¼ Teaspoon Cinnamon
- 1 Tablespoon Ginger, Fresh & Grated
- Pinch Cardamom
- 1 Tablespoon Chia Seeds
- 2 Medjool Dates, Pitted
- 1 Cup Alfalfa Sprouts
- 1 Cup Water
- 1 Banana
- ½ Cup Coconut Milk, Unsweetened

Directions:

1. Blend everything together until smooth.

35. Mango Smoothie

Preparation Time: 5 Minutes

Cooking Time: 0 minutes

Servings: 3

Ingredients:

- 1 Carrot, Peeled & Chopped
- 1 Cup Strawberries
- 1 Cup Water
- 1 Cup Peaches, Chopped
- 1 Banana, Frozen & sliced
- 1 Cup Mango, Chopped

Directions:

1. Blend everything together until smooth.

Nutrition: calories 221, fat 1, carbs 5, protein 4

36. Spinach Peach Banana Smoothie

Preparation Time: 10 minutes

Cooking Time: 0 minutes

Servings: 2

Ingredients:

- 1 cup baby spinach
- 2 cups coconut water
- 1 tablespoon agave syrup
- 2 ripe bananas
- 2 ripe peaches, pitted and chopped

Directions:

1. Add all ingredients to the blender and blend until smooth and creamy.
2. Serve immediately and enjoy.

Nutrition: calories 163, fat 1, carbs 4, protein 6

37. Salty Green Smoothie

Preparation Time: 10 minutes

Cooking Time: 0 minutes

Servings: 2

Ingredients:

- 1 cup ice cubes
- 1/4 tablespoon liquid aminos
- 1 and 1/2 tablespoon sea salt
- 2 limes, peeled and quartered
- 1 avocado, pitted and peeled
- 1 cup kale leaves
- 1 cucumber, chopped
- 2 cups tomato, chopped
- 1/4 cup water

Directions:

1. Add all ingredients to the blender and blend until smooth and creamy.
2. Serve immediately and enjoy.

Nutrition: calories 108, fat 1, carbs 1, protein 4

38. Watermelon Strawberry Smoothie

Preparation Time: 10 minutes

Cooking Time: 0 minutes

Servings: 2

Ingredients:

- 1 cup coconut milk yogurt
- 1/2 cup strawberries
- 2 cups fresh watermelon
- 1 banana

Directions:

1. Toss in all your ingredients into your blender then process until smooth.

2. Serve and Enjoy.

Nutrition: calories 160, fat 1, carbs 3, protein 4

39. Watermelon Kale Smoothie

Preparation Time: 10 minutes

Cooking Time: 0 minutes

Servings: 2

Ingredients:

- 8 oz water
- 1 orange, peeled
- 3 cups kale, chopped
- 1 banana, peeled
- 2 cups watermelon, chopped
- 1 celery, chopped

Directions:

1. Add all ingredients to the blender and blend until smooth and creamy.
2. Serve immediately and Enjoy.

Nutrition: calories 122, fat 1, carbs 5, protein 1

40. Mix Berry Watermelon Smoothie

Preparation Time: 10 minutes

Cooking Time: 0 minutes

Servings: 2

Ingredients:

- 1 cup alkaline water
- 2 fresh lemon juices
- 1/4 cup fresh mint leaves
- 1 and 1/2 cup mixed berries
- 2 cups watermelon

Directions:

1. Toss in all your ingredients into your blender then process until smooth. Serve immediately and Enjoy.

Nutrition: calories 188, fat 1, carbs 2, protein 1

41. Healthy Green Smoothie

Preparation Time: 10 minutes

Cooking Time: 0 minutes

Servings: 3

Ingredients:

- 1 cup water
- 1 fresh lemon, peeled
- 1 avocado
- 1 cucumber, peeled
- 1 cup spinach
- 1 cup ice cubes

Directions:

1. Add all ingredients to the blender and blend until smooth and creamy.
2. Serve immediately and enjoy.

Nutrition: Calories: 160, Fat 13, Carbs: 12, Protein 2

42. Apple Spinach Cucumber Smoothie

Preparation Time: 10 minutes

Cooking Time: 0 minutes

Servings: 1

Ingredients:

- 3/4 cup water
- 1/2 green apple, diced
- 3/4 cup spinach
- 1/2 cucumber

Directions:

1. Add all ingredients to the blender and blend until smooth and creamy.
2. Serve immediately and enjoy.

Nutrition: calories 90, fat 1, carbs 21, protein 1

43. Refreshing Lime Smoothie

Preparation Time: 10 minutes

Cooking Time: 0 minutes

Servings: 2

Ingredients:

- 1 cup ice cubes
- 20 drops liquid stevia
- 2 fresh lime, peeled and halved
- 1 tablespoon lime zest, grated
- 1/2 cucumber, chopped
- 1 avocado, pitted and peeled
- 2 cups spinach
- 1 tablespoon creamed coconut
- 3/4 cup coconut water

Directions:

1. Add all ingredients to the blender and blend until smooth and creamy.
2. Serve immediately and enjoy.

Nutrition: calories 312, fat 3, carbs 28, protein 4

44. Broccoli Green Smoothie

Preparation Time: 10 minutes

Cooking Time: 0 minutes

Servings: 2

Ingredients:

- 1 celery, peeled and chopped
- 1 lemon, peeled
- 1 apple, diced
- 1 banana
- 1 cup spinach
- 1/2 cup broccoli

Directions:

1. Add all ingredients to the blender and blend until smooth and creamy.
2. Serve immediately and enjoy.

Nutrition: calories 121, fat 1, carbs 18, protein 1

45. Healthy Vegetable Smoothie

Preparation Time: 10 minutes

Cooking Time: 0 minutes

Servings: 2

Ingredients:

- 1 cup ice cubes
- 2 cups fresh spinach
- 2 celery stalks
- 1/2 cup fresh parsley
- 1 cucumber
- 1 lemon juice
- 1 avocado

Directions:

1. Add all ingredients to the blender and blend until smooth and creamy.
2. Serve immediately and enjoy.

Nutrition: calories 210, fat 3, carbs 17, protein 11

46. Refreshing Green Smoothie

Preparation Time: 10 minutes

Cooking Time: 0 minutes

Servings: 2

Ingredients:

- 1 cup ice cubes
- 1/2 lemon juice
- 1/2 cucumber, chopped
- 1/4 cup parsley
- 1 cup spinach
- 1/2 cup water
- 1/4 cup peaches, sliced
- 1 banana

Directions:

1. Add all ingredients to the blender and blend until smooth and creamy.
2. Serve immediately and enjoy.

Nutrition: calories 90, fat 1, carbs 20, protein

47. Sweet Green Smoothie

Preparation Time: 10 minutes

Cooking Time: 0 minutes

Servings: 1

Ingredients:

- 2 tablespoons flax seeds
- 1/2 cup wheatgrass
- 1 mango
- 1 cup pomegranate juice

Directions:

1. Add all ingredients to the blender and blend until smooth and creamy.
2. Serve immediately and enjoy.

Nutrition: calories 177, fat 1, carbs 21, protein 5

48. Avocado Mango Smoothie

Preparation Time: 10 minutes

Cooking Time: 0 minutes

Servings: 2

Ingredients:

- 1 cup ice cubes
- 1/2 cup mango
- 1/2 avocado
- 1 tablespoon ginger
- 3 kale leaves
- 1 cup coconut water

Directions:

1. Toss in all your ingredients into your blender then process until smooth.
2. Serve and Enjoy.

Nutrition: calories 290, fat 3, carbs 18, protein 11

49. Super Healthy Green Smoothie

Preparation Time: 10 minutes

Cooking Time: 0 minutes

Servings: 2

Ingredients:

- 1 teaspoon spirulina powder
- 1 cup coconut water
- 2 cups mixed greens
- 1 tablespoon ginger
- 4 tablespoon lemon juice
- 2 celery stalks
- 1 cup cucumber, chopped
- 1 green pear, core removed

- 1 banana

Directions:

1. Add all ingredients to the blender and blend until smooth and creamy.
2. Serve immediately and enjoy.

Nutrition: calories 161, fat 1, carbs 19, protein 7

50. Spinach Coconut Smoothie

Preparation Time: 10 minutes

Cooking Time: 0 minutes

Servings: 2

Ingredients:

- 2 tablespoons unsweetened coconut flakes
- 2 cups fresh pineapple
- 1/2 cup coconut water
- 1 and 1/2 cups coconut milk
- 2 cups fresh spinach

Directions:

1. Add all ingredients to the blender and blend until smooth and creamy.
2. Serve immediately and enjoy.

Nutrition: calories 290, fat 1, carbs 22, protein 8

51. Pear Kale Smoothie

Preparation Time: 10 minutes

Cooking Time: 0 minutes

Servings: 2

Ingredients:

- 1 cup apple juice
- 1 cup water
- 1/4 cup mint leaves
- 2 cups kale

- 1 ripe pear, cored and chopped

Directions:

1. Add all ingredients to the blender and blend until smooth and creamy.
2. Serve immediately and enjoy.

Nutrition: calories 130, fat 1, carbs 18, protein 3

52. Banana Peach Smoothie

Preparation Time: 10 minutes

Cooking Time: 0 minutes

Servings: 2

Ingredients:

- 1 cup coconut water
- 1 teaspoon agave syrup
- 1 and 1/4 oz spinach
- 1 banana
- 1 ripe peach

Directions:

1. Add all ingredients to the blender and blend until smooth and creamy.
2. Serve immediately and enjoy.

Nutrition: calories 120, fat 2, carbs 28, protein 10

53. Refreshing Alkaline Smoothie

Preparation Time: 10 minutes

Cooking Time: 0 minutes

Servings: 2

Ingredients:

- 1/2 cup ice cubes
- 1 tbsp ginger
- 1/4 cup fresh mint leaves
- 1/2 cup parsley

- 1 cucumber, chopped
- 1 lemon juice
- 1 cup water
- 4 cups baby spinach
- 1 avocado

Directions:

1. Add all ingredients to the blender and blend until smooth and creamy.
2. Serve immediately and enjoy.

Nutrition: calories 267, fat 1, carbs 10, protein 4

54. Coconut Celery Smoothie

Preparation Time: 10 minutes

Cooking Time: 0 minutes

Servings: 2

Ingredients:

- 3 celeries, shredded
- 1 teaspoon ground cinnamon
- 1/2 banana
- 1 scoop protein powder
- 1 tablespoon coconut butter
- 1 cup unsweetened coconut milk

Directions:

1. Add all ingredients to the blender and blend until smooth and creamy.
2. Serve immediately and enjoy.

Nutrition: calories 319, fat 1, carbs 18, protein 9

55. Blueberry Coconut Smoothie

Preparation Time: 10 minutes

Cooking Time: 0 minutes

Servings: 1

Ingredients:

- 1 tablespoon hemp seeds
- 1/2 cup blueberries
- 1 teaspoon ground cinnamon
- 1/2 banana
- 1 scoop protein powder
- 1 tablespoon coconut butter
- 1 cup unsweetened coconut milk

Directions:

1. Add all ingredients to the blender and blend until smooth and creamy.
2. Serve immediately and enjoy.

Nutrition: calories 211, fat 1, carbs 19, protein 8

56. Kiwi Cucumber Boosting Smoothie

Preparation Time: 10 minutes

Cooking Time: 0 minutes

Servings: 1

Ingredients:

- 1 cup spinach
- 1 cup ice cubes
- 1 kiwi fruit
- 1/2 banana
- 1/4 cucumber
- 1/4 cup coconut milk

Directions:

1. Add all ingredients to the blender and blend until smooth and creamy.
2. Serve immediately and enjoy.

Nutrition: calories 255, fat 1, carbs 20, protein 6

57. Spinach Protein Smoothie

Preparation Time: 10 minutes

Cooking Time: 0 minutes

Servings: 2

Ingredients:

- 1 and 1/2 cups unsweetened coconut milk
- 1/2 cup yogurt
- 1/2 teaspoon cinnamon
- 1 tablespoon protein powder
- 1/2 banana
- 2 cups spinach

Directions:

1. Toss in all your ingredients into your blender then process until smooth.
2. Serve and enjoy.

Nutrition: calories 390, fat 1, carbs 24, protein 11

58. Tropical Smoothie

Preparation Time: 10 minutes

Cooking Time: 0 minutes

Servings: 1

Ingredients:

- 1/4 cup coconut water
- 1/2 cup yogurt
- 1 tablespoon honey
- 2 tablespoons shredded coconut

- 1/2 cup mango
- 1/2 cup pineapple
- 1 and 1/2 cup spinach

Directions:

1. Add all ingredients to the blender and blend until smooth and creamy.
2. Serve immediately and enjoy.

Nutrition: calories 219, fat 1, carbs 9, protein 4

59. Berry Kale Smoothie

Preparation Time: 10 minutes

Cooking Time: 0 minutes

Servings: 1

Ingredients:

- 1 cup orange juice
- 1/2 cup yogurt
- 1 banana
- 1/4 cup raspberries
- 1/2 cup strawberries
- 1 cup kale

Directions:

1. Add all ingredients to the blender and blend until smooth and creamy.
2. Serve immediately and enjoy.

Nutrition: calories 312, fat 2, carbs 18, protein 12

60. Basil Kale Strawberry Smoothie

Preparation Time: 10 minutes

Cooking Time: 0 minutes

Servings: 2

Ingredients:

- 1 and 1/2 cups unsweetened coconut milk
- 1 tablespoon flax seeds
- 1/4 cup basil
- 3 strawberries
- 1/2 banana
- 1 cup kale

Directions:

1. Add all ingredients to the blender and blend until smooth and creamy.
2. Serve immediately and enjoy.

Nutrition: calories 203, fat 3, carbs 28, protein 5

61. Chia Strawberry Smoothie

Preparation Time: 10 minutes

Cooking Time: 0 minutes

Servings: 2

Ingredients:

- 4 drops liquid stevia
- 1/2 lemon juice
- 1/2 small beetroot, chopped
- 1 cup strawberries
- 4 romaine lettuce leaves, chopped
- 2 celery stalks, chopped
- 2 tablespoons chia seeds
- 1 cup coconut water

Directions:

1. Add all ingredients to the blender and blend until smooth and creamy.
2. Serve immediately and enjoy.

Nutrition: calories 90, fat 3, carbs 15, protein 3

62. Strawberry Banana Smoothie

Preparation Time: 10 minutes

Cooking Time: 0 minutes

Servings: 1

Ingredients:

- 1 cup unsweetened coconut milk
- 1 banana
- 1/2 cup strawberries

Directions:

1. Add all ingredients to the blender and blend until smooth and creamy.
2. Serve immediately and enjoy.

Nutrition: calories 85, fat 3, carbs 18, protein 11

63. Easy Mango Lassi

Preparation Time: 10 minutes

Cooking Time: 0 minutes

Servings: 4

Ingredients

- 2 cups plain whole-milk yogurt
- 1 cup milk
- 3 mangoes - peeled, seeded, and chopped
- 4 tsps. white sugar, or to taste
- 1/8 tsp. ground cardamom

Directions:

1. In the jar of a blender, place cardamom, white sugar, mangoes, milk, and yogurt.
2. Blend together for about 2 minutes or until smooth.
3. Chill in the refrigerator until cold, about 1 hour.
4. Serve with a small sprinkling of ground cardamom.

Nutrition: calories 220, fat 1, carbs 24, protein 4

64. Holly Goodness Smoothie

Preparation Time: 10 minutes

Cooking Time: 0 minutes

Servings: 1

Ingredients

- 1 mango - peeled, seeded, and chopped
- 1 small banana
- 1/2 cup frozen raspberries
- 1/2 cup almond milk
- 1/2 cup hemp milk
- 1 tsp. vanilla extract
- 1 tsp. chia seeds
- 1 tsp. hemp seeds
- 1 tsp. maca powder

Directions:

1. Blend together maca powder, hemp seeds, chia seeds, vanilla extract, hemp milk, almond milk, raspberries, banana, and mango using a blender until the mixture is smooth.

Nutrition: calories 380, fat 2, carbs 20, protein 11

65. Honey-mango Smoothie

Preparation Time: 10 minutes

Cooking Time: 0 minutes

Servings: 2

Ingredients:

- 1 mango - peeled, seeded, and cubed
- 1 tbsp. white sugar
- 2 tbsps. honey
- 1 cup nonfat milk
- 1 tsp. lemon juice

- 1 cup ice cubes

Directions:

1. In a blender pitcher, put sugar, honey, and mango; add lemon juice and milk, conflate till smooth. Distribute ice cubes among 2 serving glasses.
2. Put mango smoothie on ice and serve.

Nutrition: calories 310, fat 3, carbs 28, protein 3

66. Hong Kong Mango Drink

Preparation Time: 10 minutes

Cooking Time: 0 minutes

Servings: 2

Ingredients:

- 1/2 cup small pearl tapioca
- 1 mango - peeled, seeded, and diced
- 14 ice cubes
- 1/2 cup coconut milk

Directions:

1. Over high heat, boil water.
2. When the water is boiling, mix in the tapioca pearls then boil again.
3. Uncover while cooking the tapioca pearls for 10 minutes, mixing from time to time. Put the cover back then take off heat, let it rest for half an hour.
4. In a colander placed in the sink, drain well; cover then chill.
5. In a blender, blend ice and mango till smooth. In 2 tall glasses, distribute chilled tapioca pearls; pour the mango mixture on top then pour on top of each with a quarter cup coconut milk.

Nutrition: calories 324, fat 2, carbs 21, protein 9

67. Jack-o'-lantern Smoothie Bowl

Preparation Time: 10 minutes

Cooking Time: 0 minutes

Servings: 1

Ingredients:

- 1 cup frozen mango chunks
- ¾ cup reduced-fat plain Greek yogurt
- ¼ cup reduced-fat milk
- 1 tsp. vanilla extract
- 1 strawberry, hulled and halved
- 1 tsp. chia seeds

Directions:

1. In a blender, combine vanilla, milk, yogurt, and mango.
2. Puree the mixture until smooth.
3. Pour the entire smoothie into a bowl and decorate to make the drink look like a jack-o-lantern.
4. Use halved strawberries to make the cheeks and use the chia seeds to make eyes and a nose.
5. Serve the smoothie with a green spoon attached with a paper leaf to make it look like a pumpkin stem.

Nutrition: calories 186, fat 1, carbs 18, protein 9

Chapter 8

SALAD AND SOUPS

68. Coconut Watercress Soup

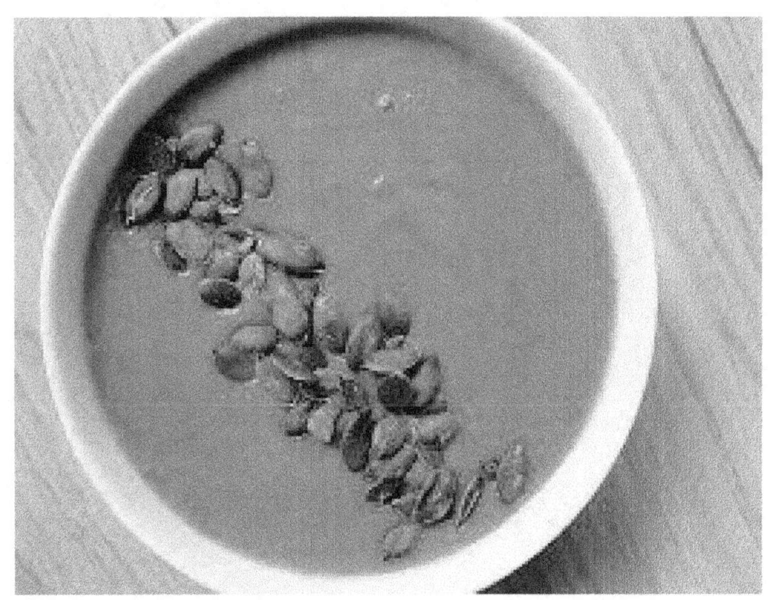

Preparation time: 10 minutes

Cooking time: 20 minutes

Servings: 4

Ingredients:

- 1 teaspoon coconut oil
- 1 onion, diced
- ¾ cup coconut milk

Directions:

1. Preparing the ingredients.
2. Melt the coconut oil in a large pot over medium-high heat. Add the onion and cook until soft, about 5 minutes, then add the peas and the water. Bring to a boil, then lower the heat and add the watercress, mint, salt, and pepper.
3. Cover and simmer for 5 minutes. Stir in the coconut milk and purée the soup until smooth in a blender or with an immersion blender.
4. Try this soup with any other fresh, leafy green—anything from spinach to collard greens to arugula to swiss chard.

Nutrition: calories 170, fat 3, carbs 18, protein 6

69. Roasted Red Pepper and Butternut Squash Soup

Preparation time: 10 minutes

Cooking time: 45 minutes

Servings: 6

Ingredients:

- 1 small butternut squash
- 1 tablespoon olive oil
- 1 teaspoon sea salt
- 2 red bell peppers
- 1 yellow onion
- 1 head garlic
- 2 cups water, or vegetable broth
- Zest and juice of 1 lime
- 1 to 2 tablespoons tahini
- Pinch cayenne pepper
- ½ teaspoon ground coriander
- ½ teaspoon ground cumin
- Toasted squash seeds (optional)

Directions:

1. Preparing the ingredients.

2. Preheat the oven to 350°f.

3. Prepare the squash for roasting by cutting it in half lengthwise, scooping out the seeds, and poking some holes in the flesh with a fork. Reserve the seeds if desired.

4. Rub a small amount of oil over the flesh and skin, then rub with a bit of sea salt and put the halves skin-side down in a large baking dish. Put it in the oven while you prepare the rest of the vegetables.

5. Prepare the peppers the exact same way, except they do not need to be poked.

6. Slice the onion in half and rub oil on the exposed faces. Slice the top off the head of garlic and rub oil on the exposed flesh.

7. After the squash has cooked for 20 minutes, add the peppers, onion, and garlic, and roast for another 20 minutes. Optionally, you can toast the squash seeds by putting them in the oven in a separate baking dish 10 to 15 minutes before the vegetables are finished.

8. Keep a close eye on them. When the vegetables are cooked, take them out and let them cool before handling them. The squash will be very soft when poked with a fork.

9. Scoop the flesh out of the squash skin into a large pot (if you have an immersion blender) or into a blender.

10. Chop the pepper roughly, remove the onion skin and chop the onion roughly, and squeeze the garlic cloves out of the head, all into the pot or blender. Add the water, the lime zest and juice, and the tahini. Purée the soup, adding more water if you like, to your desired consistency. Season with salt, cayenne, coriander, and cumin. Serve garnished with toasted squash seeds (if using).

Nutrition: calories 150, fat 3, carbs 20, protein 6

70. Tomato Pumpkin Soup

Preparation time: 25 minutes

Cooking time: 15 minutes

Servings: 4

Ingredients:

- 2 cups pumpkin, diced
- 1/2 cup tomato, chopped
- 1/2 cup onion, chopped
- 1 1/2 tsp curry powder
- 1/2 tsp paprika
- 2 cups vegetable stock
- 1 tsp olive oil
- 1/2 tsp garlic, minced

Directions:

1. In a saucepan, add oil, garlic, and onion and sauté for 3 minutes over medium heat.
2. Add remaining ingredients into the saucepan and bring to boil.
3. Reduce heat and cover and simmer for 10 minutes.
4. Puree the soup using a blender until smooth.
5. Stir well and serve warm.

Nutrition: calories 70, fat 3, carbs 13, protein 1

71. Cauliflower Spinach Soup

Preparation time: 45 minutes

Cooking time: 25 minutes

Servings: 5

Ingredients:

- 1/2 cup unsweetened coconut milk
- 5 oz fresh spinach, chopped
- 5 watercress, chopped

- 8 cups vegetable stock
- 1 lb. cauliflower, chopped
- Salt

Directions:

1. Add stock and cauliflower in a large saucepan and bring to boil over medium heat for 15 minutes.
2. Add spinach and watercress and cook for another 10 minutes.
3. Remove from heat and puree the soup using a blender until smooth.
4. Add coconut milk and stir well. Season with salt.
5. Stir well and serve hot.

Nutrition: calories 150, fat 4, carbs 8, protein 11

72. Avocado Mint Soup

Preparation time: 10 minutes

Cooking time: 10 minutes

Servings: 2

Ingredients:

- 1 medium avocado, peeled, pitted, and cut into pieces
- 1 cup coconut milk
- 2 romaine lettuce leaves
- 20 fresh mint leaves
- 1 tbsp fresh lime juice
- 1/8 tsp salt

Directions:

1. Add all ingredients into the blender and blend until smooth. The soup should be thick not as a puree.
2. Pour into the serving bowls and place in the refrigerator for 10 minutes.
3. Stir well and serve chilled.

Nutrition: calories 290, fat 3, carbs 18, protein 11

73. Creamy Squash Soup

Preparation time: 35 minutes

Cooking time: 22 minutes

Servings: 8

Ingredients:

- 3 cups butternut squash, chopped
- 1 ½ cups unsweetened coconut milk
- 1 tbsp coconut oil
- 1 tsp dried onion flakes
- 1 tbsp curry powder
- 4 cups water
- 1 garlic clove
- 1 tsp kosher salt

Directions:

1. Add squash, coconut oil, onion flakes, curry powder, water, garlic, and salt into a large saucepan. Bring to boil over high heat.
2. Turn heat to medium and simmer for 20 minutes.
3. Puree the soup using a blender until smooth. Return soup to the saucepan and stir in coconut milk and cook for 2 minutes.
4. Stir well and serve hot.

Nutrition: calories 140, fat 2, carbs 9, protein 1

74. Alkaline Carrot Soup with Fresh Mushrooms

Preparation Time: 10 minutes

Cooking Time: 20 minutes

Servings: 1-2

Ingredients:

- 4 mid-sized carrots
- 4 mid-sized potatoes
- 10 enormous new mushrooms (champignons or chanterelles)

- 1/2 white onion
- 2 tbsp. olive oil (cold squeezed, additional virgin)
- 3 cups vegetable stock
- 2 tbsp. parsley, new and cleaved
- Salt and new white pepper

Directions:

1. Wash and strip carrots and potatoes and dice them.
2. Warm-up vegetable stock in a pot on medium heat. Cook carrots and potatoes for around 15 minutes. Meanwhile finely shape onion and braise them in a container with olive oil for around 3 minutes.
3. Wash the mushrooms, slice them to the desired size, and add to the container, cooking for an additional of approximately 5 minutes, blending at times. Blend carrots, vegetable stock, and potatoes, and put the substance of the skillet into the pot.
4. When nearly done, season with parsley, salt, and pepper and serve hot. Appreciate this alkalizing soup!

Nutrition: calories 176, fat 2, carbs 23, protein 9

75. Swiss Cauliflower-Emmental-Soup

Preparation Time: 10 minutes

Cooking Time: 15 minutes

Servings: 3-4

Ingredients:

- 2 cups cauliflower pieces
- 1 cup potatoes, cubed
- 2 cups vegetable stock (without yeast)
- 3 tbsp. Swiss Emmental cheddar, cubed
- 2 tbsp. new chives
- 1 tbsp. pumpkin seeds
- 1 touch of nutmeg and cayenne pepper

Directions:

1. Cook cauliflower and potato in vegetable stock until delicate and blend it.
2. Season the soup with nutmeg and cayenne, and possibly somewhat salt and pepper.
3. Include cheddar and chives and mix a couple of moments until the soup is smooth and prepared to serve. Enhance it with pumpkin seeds.

Nutrition: calories 89, fat 1, carbs 18, protein 9

76. Chilled Parsley-Gazpacho with Lime & Cucumber

Preparation Time: 10 minutes

Cooking Time: 2 hours

Servings: 1

Ingredients:

- 4-5 middle-sized tomatoes
- 2 tbsp. olive oil, extra virgin, and cold-pressed
- 2 large cups fresh parsley
- 2 ripe avocados
- 2 cloves garlic, diced
- 2 limes, juiced
- 4 cups vegetable broth
- 1 middle-sized cucumber
- 2 small red onions, diced
- 1 tsp. dried oregano
- 1½ tsp. paprika powder
- ½ tsp. cayenne pepper
- Sea salt and freshly ground pepper to taste

Directions:

1. In a pan, heat up olive oil and sauté onions and garlic until translucent. Set aside to cool down.
2. Use a large blender and blend parsley, avocado, tomatoes, cucumber, vegetable broth, lime juice, and onion-garlic mix until smooth. Add some

water if desired, and season with cayenne pepper, paprika powder, oregano, salt, and pepper. Blend again and put in the fridge for at least 1, 5 hours.

Nutrition: calories 156, fat 1, carbs 24, protein 9

77. Chilled Avocado Tomato Soup

Preparation Time: 7 minutes

Cooking Time: 20 minutes

Servings: 1-2

Ingredients:

- 2 small avocados
- 2 large tomatoes
- 1 stalk of celery
- 1 small onion
- 1 clove of garlic
- Juice of 1 fresh lemon
- 1 cup of water (best: alkaline water)
- A handful of fresh lavages
- Parsley and sea salt to taste

Directions:

1. Scoop the avocados and cut all veggies into little pieces.
2. Spot all fixings in a blender and blend until smooth.
3. Serve chilled and appreciate this nutritious and sound soluble soup formula!

Nutrition: calories 210, fat 1, carbs 18, protein 9

78. Pumpkin and White Bean Soup with Sage

Preparation Time: 10 minutes

Cooking Time: 40 minutes

Servings: 3-4

Ingredients:

- 1 ½ pound pumpkin
- ½ pound yams
- ½ pound white beans
- 1 onion
- 2 cloves of garlic
- 1 tbsp. of cold squeezed additional virgin olive oil
- 1 tbsp. of spices (your top picks)
- 1 tbsp. of sage
- 1 ½ quart water (best: antacid water)
- A spot of ocean salt and pepper

Directions:

1. Cut the pumpkin and potatoes in shapes, cut the onion, and cut the garlic, the spices, and the sage in fine pieces.
2. Sauté the onion and also the garlic in olive oil for around two or three minutes.
3. Include the potatoes, pumpkin, spices, and sage and fry for an additional 5 minutes.
4. At that point include the water and cook for around 30 minutes (spread the pot with a top) until vegetables are delicate.
5. At long last include the beans and some salt and pepper. Cook for an additional 5 minutes and serve right away. Prepared!! Appreciate this antacid soup. Alkalizing tasty!

Nutrition: calories 218, fat 1, carbs 11, protein 8

79. Alkaline Carrot Soup with Millet

Preparation Time: 7 minutes

Cooking Time: 40 minutes

Servings: 3-4

Ingredients:

- 2 cups cauliflower pieces
- 1 cup potatoes, cubed

- 2 cups vegetable stock (without yeast)
- 3 tbsp. Swiss Emmental cheddar, cubed
- 2 tbsp. new chives
- 1 tbsp. pumpkin seeds
- 1 touch of nutmeg and cayenne pepper

Directions:

1. Cook cauliflower and potato in vegetable stock until delicate and blend it.
2. Season the soup with nutmeg and cayenne, and possibly somewhat salt and pepper.
3. Include Emmental cheddar and chives and mix a couple of moments until the soup is smooth and prepared to serve. It can be enhanced with pumpkin seeds.

Nutrition: calories 90, fat 1, carbs 18, protein 11

80. Alkaline Pumpkin Tomato Soup

Preparation Time: 15 minutes

Cooking Time: 30 minutes

Servings: 3-4

Ingredients:

- 1 quart of water (if accessible: soluble water)
- 400g new tomatoes, stripped and diced
- 1 medium-sized sweet pumpkin
- 5 yellow onions
- 1 tbsp. cold squeezed additional virgin olive oil
- 2 tsp. ocean salt or natural salt
- Touch of cayenne pepper
- Your preferred spices (discretionary)
- Bunch of new parsley

Directions:

1. Cut onions in little pieces and sauté with some oil in a significant pot.
2. Cut the pumpkin down the middle, at that point remove the stem and scoop out the seeds.
3. At long last scoop out the fragile living creature and put it in the pot.
4. Include likewise the tomatoes and the water and cook for around 20 minutes.
5. At that point empty the soup into a food processor and blend well for a couple of moments. Sprinkle with salt, pepper, and other spices.
6. Fill bowls and trimming with new parsley. Make the most of your alkalizing soup!

Nutrition: calories 190, fat 3, carbs 18, protein 11

81. Alkaline Pumpkin Coconut Soup

Preparation Time: 10 minutes

Cooking Time: 15 minutes

Servings: 3-4

Ingredients:

- 2 lb pumpkin
- 6 cups of water (best: soluble water delivered with a water ionizer)
- 1 cup low-fat coconut milk
- 5 ounces of potatoes
- 2 major onions
- 3 ounces leek
- 1 bunch of new parsley
- 1 touch of nutmeg
- 1 touch of cayenne pepper
- 1 tsp. ocean salt or natural salt
- 4 tbsp. cold squeezed additional virgin olive oil

Directions:

1. As a matter of first significance: cut the onions, the pumpkin, and the potatoes just as the hole into little pieces.

2. At that point, heat the olive oil in a significant pot and sauté the onions for a couple of moments.
3. At that point, include the water and heat up the pumpkin, potatoes, and the leek until delicate.
4. Include coconut milk.
5. Presently utilize a hand blender and puree for around 1 moment. The soup should turn out to be extremely velvety.
6. Season with salt, pepper, and nutmeg. Lastly, include the parsley and appreciate this alkalizing pumpkin soup hot or cold!

Nutrition: calories 90, fat 3, carbs 23, protein 1

82. Cold Cauliflower-Coconut Soup

Preparation Time: 7 minutes

Cooking Time: 20 minutes

Servings: 3-4

Ingredients:

- 1 pound (450g) new cauliflower
- 1 ¼ cup (300ml) unsweetened coconut milk
- 1 cup of water (best: antacid water)
- 2 tbsp. new lime juice
- 1/3 cup cold squeezed additional virgin olive oil
- 1 cup new coriander leaves, slashed
- Spot of salt and cayenne pepper
- 1 bunch of unsweetened coconut chips

Directions:

1. Steam cauliflower for around 10 minutes.
2. At that point, set up the cauliflower with coconut milk and water in a food processor and get it started until extremely smooth.
3. Include new lime squeeze, salt and pepper, a large portion of the cleaved coriander, and the oil and blend for an additional couple of moments.
4. Pour in soup bowls and embellishment with coriander and coconut chips. Enjoy!

Nutrition: calories 190, fat 1, carbs 21, protein 6

83. Raw Avocado-Broccoli Soup with Cashew Nuts

Preparation Time: 10 minutes

Cooking Time: 30 minutes

Servings: 1-2

Ingredients:

- ½ cup of water (if available: alkaline water)
- ½ avocado
- 1 cup chopped broccoli
- ½ cup cashew nuts
- ½ cup alfalfa sprouts
- 1 clove of garlic
- 1 tbsp. cold-pressed extra virgin olive oil
- 1 pinch of sea salt and pepper
- Some parsley to garnish

Directions:

1. Put the cashew nuts in a blender or food processor, include some water and puree for a couple of moments.
2. Include the various fixings (except for the avocado) individually and puree each an ideal opportunity for a couple of moments.
3. Dispense the soup in a container and warm it up to the normal room temperature. Enhance with salt and pepper. In the interim dice the avocado and slash the parsley.
4. Dispense the soup in a container or plate; include the avocado slices and embellishment with parsley.
5. That's it! Enjoy this excellent healthy soup!

Nutrition: calories 48, fat 1, carbs 21, protein 8

84. Chilled Cucumber and Lime Soup

Preparation Time: 5 minutes

Cooking Time: 20 minutes

Servings: 1-2

Chilled soups are perfect for the hot summer months, and this easy soup is made with garden fresh vegetables with no cooking involved. Simply prepare the veggies, add them to a blender, and lunch is served!

Ingredients:

- 1 cucumber, peeled
- ½ zucchini, peeled
- 1 tablespoon freshly squeezed lime juice
- 1 tablespoon fresh cilantro leaves
- 1 garlic clove, crushed
- ¼ teaspoon of sea salt

Directions:

1. In a blender, blend the cucumber, zucchini, lime juice, cilantro, garlic, and salt until well combined. Add more salt, if necessary.
2. Fill 1 huge or 2 little dishes and enjoy immediately or refrigerate for 15 to 20 minutes to chill before serving.

Nutrition: calories 90, fat 1, carbs 12, protein 5

85. Lime & Mint Summer Fruit Salad

Preparation Time: 10 minutes

Cooking Time: 0 minutes

Serving: 4

Ingredients:

- ¼ cup apple, peeled and diced
- ¼ cup grapes
- 2 tablespoons mint, fresh and chopped
- 2 tablespoons Seville orange juice, freshly squeezed

- ¼ cup strawberries
- ¼ cup peaches, peeled and diced
- ¼ cup tangerine slices
- ¼ cup cantaloupe, small bite-size pieces
- ¼ cup honeydew melon, small bite-size pieces
- ¼ cup watermelon, small bite-size pieces

Directions:

1. In a mixing bowl, combine all of the fruit.
2. Add the Seville orange juice, mint, and mix well.
3. Serve chilled and enjoy!

Nutrition: calories 185, fat 1, carbs 18, protein 1

86. Cherry Tomato & Kale Salad

Preparation Time: 10 minutes

Cooking Time: 0 minutes

Serving: 2

Ingredients:

- 2 tbsps. Ranch dressing
- 2 cups organic baby tomatoes
- 1 bunch kale, stemmed, leaves washed and chopped

Directions:

1. Mix all the ingredients in a bowl.
2. Divide the salad equally into two serving dishes.
3. Serve.

Nutrition: calories 116, fat 1, carbs 12, protein 8

87. Radish Noodle Salad

Preparation Time: 10 minutes

Cooking Time: 0 minutes

Serving: 4

Ingredients:

- 2 cups cooked radish florets
- 1 roasted spaghetti squash
- 1 chopped scallion
- 1 tbsp. sesame oil
- 1 bell seeded pepper, cut into strips
- 2 tbsps. Toasted sesame seeds
- 1 tsp. sea salt
- 1 tsp. red pepper flakes

Directions:

1. Start by preparing the spaghetti squash by removing the cooked squash with a fork into a bowl.
2. Add the radish, red bell pepper, and scallion to the bowl with the squash.
3. In a small bowl, mix the red pepper flakes, salt, and sesame oil.
4. Drizzle the mixture to top the vegetables. Toss gently to combine them.
5. Add the sesame seeds to garnish.
6. Serve.

Nutrition: calories 112, fat 1, carbs 8, protein 2

88. Caprese Salad

Preparation Time: 5 minutes

Cooking Time: 0 minutes

Serving: 2

Ingredients:

- 1 sliced avocado
- 2 sliced large tomatoes
- 1 bunch basil leaves
- 1 tsp. sea salt
- 1 cup cubed jackfruit

Directions:

1. In a bowl toss all the salad ingredients to mix.
2. Add the sea salt to season.
3. Serve.

Nutrition: calories 125, fat 1, carbs 18, protein 3

89. Summer Lettuce Salad

Preparation Time: 5 minutes

Cooking Time: 0 minutes

Serving: 4

Ingredients:

- 2 cups halved cherry tomatoes
- 4 cups romaine lettuce or iceberg
- 1 peeled and sliced cucumber
- 2 thinly sliced radishes
- 1 sliced scallion
- 1/2 cup shredded zucchini
- 14 oz. can drained whole green beans

Directions:

1. Add all of the salad ingredients in a large bowl then toss with 2 tbsps. Of the dressing.
2. Serve.

Nutrition: calories 143, fat 1, carbs 12, protein 1

90. Mustard Cabbage Salad

Preparation Time: 10 Minutes

Cooking Time: 0

Servings: 4

Ingredients:

- 1 green cabbage head, shredded
- 1 red cabbage head, shredded
- 2 tablespoons avocado oil
- 2 tablespoons mustard
- 1 tablespoon balsamic vinegar
- 1 teaspoon hot paprika
- Salt and black pepper to the taste
- 1 tablespoon dill, chopped

Directions:

1. In a bowl, mix the cabbage with the oil, mustard, and the other ingredients, toss, divide between plates and serve as a side salad.

Nutrition: calories 150, fat 1, carbs 6, protein 3

91. Alkaline-Electric Spring Salad

Preparation Time: 11 minutes

Cooking Time: 15 Minutes

Serving: 2

Ingredients

- 1 cup cherry tomatoes
- 4 cups seasonal greens
- 1/4 cup walnuts
- 1/4 cup approved herbs
- For the dressing:
- Sea salt and cayenne pepper
- 3 key limes
- 1 tablespoon of homemade raw sesame tahini butter

Directions:

1. Sap the key limes.
2. Whisk together the homemade raw sesame "tahini" butter with the key lime juice in a small bowl.

3. Add cayenne pepper and sea salt to your satisfaction.
4. Cut the cherry tomatoes in half.
5. In a large bowl, combine the greens, cherry tomatoes, and herbs. Pour the dressing on top and massage with your hands.
6. Let the greens soak the dressing. Add more cayenne pepper, herbs, and sea salt.
7. Enjoy

Nutrition: calories 218, fat 1, carbs 19, protein 2

92. Super Healthy Beet Greens Salad

Preparation Time: 10 Minutes

Cooking Time: 0

Servings: 4

Ingredients:

For Dressing:

- 1 garlic clove, minced
- 1 ½ teaspoons of Dijon mustard
- 3 tablespoons of extra-virgin olive oil
- 1 tablespoon balsamic vinegar
- Salt and freshly ground black pepper, to taste
- 2 cups of vegetable broth
- ¼ cup of olive oil

For Salad:

- 8 cup of fresh beet greens
- ¼ cup of feta cheese, crumbled

Directions:

1. Prepare dressing in a bowl by adding all the dressing ingredients and beat until well combined.
2. In a large bowl, mix together greens and cheese.
3. Pour dressing over salad and toss to coat well. Serve immediately.

Nutrition: calories 250, fat 1, carbs 19, protein 1

93. Super Delicious Cucumber Salad

Preparation Time: 10 Minutes

Cooking Time: 0

Servings: 8

Ingredients:

- ½ cup of sour cream
- 1 teaspoon of white vinegar
- ½ teaspoon of powdered stevia
- ½ teaspoon of dill weed
- Salt, to taste
- 4 medium cucumbers, sliced

Directions:

1. In a bowl, add all the ingredients except cucumbers and beat until well combined.
2. Add cucumber slices and stir until well combined.
3. Refrigerate to chill for at least 30 minutes before serving.

Nutrition: calories 84, fat 1, carbs 10, protein 1

94. Nutty and Fruity Garden Salad

Preparation time: 10 minutes

Cooking time: 0 minutes

Servings: 2

Ingredients:

- 6 cups baby spinach
- ½ cup chopped walnuts, toasted
- 1 ripe red pear, sliced
- 1 ripe persimmon, sliced
- 1 teaspoon garlic minced
- 1 shallot, minced
- 1 tablespoon extra-virgin olive oil

- 2 tablespoons fresh lemon juice
- 1 teaspoon wholegrain mustard

Directions:

1. Mix well garlic, shallot, oil, lemon juice, and mustard in a large salad bowl.
2. Add spinach, pear, and persimmon. Toss to coat well.
3. To serve, garnish with chopped pecans.

Nutrition: calories 330, fat 1, carbs 18, protein 1

95. A Snowy "Frozen" Salad Bowl

Preparation Time: 75 Minutes

Cooking Time: 0

Servings: 3

Ingredients:

- ½ a cup of white sugar
- 2 cups of water
- 1 can of 20-ounce frozen orange juice concentrate (thawed)
- 1 can of 20-ounce frozen lemonade concentrated (thawed)
- 4 bananas, sliced
- 1 can have crushed pineapple (with juice)
- 1 pack of strawberries (thawed)

Directions:

1. Take a bowl and add water and sugar
2. Dissolve the sugar and add orange juice, bananas, lemonade, crushed pineapples (alongside the juice), and strawberries and give it a nice mix
3. Pour the mixture into a 9x13 inch glass pan and allow it to chill
4. Once ready to serve, let it sit for about 5 minutes at room temp and cut them out

Nutrition: calories 210, fat 1, carbs 21, protein 1

96. Warm Mushroom and Orange Pepper Salad

Preparation Time: 10 Minutes

Cooking Time: 8 Minutes

Servings: 4

Ingredients:

- 2 tbsp. avocado oil
- 1 cup mixed mushrooms, chopped
- 2 orange bell peppers, deseeded and finely sliced
- 1 garlic clove, minced
- 2 tbsp. tamarind sauce
- 1 tsp. maple (sugar-free) syrup
- ½ tsp. hot sauce
- ½ tsp. fresh ginger paste
- Sesame seeds to garnish

Directions:

1. Over medium fire, heat half of avocado oil in a large skillet, sauté mushroom, and bell peppers until slightly softened, 5 minutes.
2. In a small bowl, whisk garlic, tamarind sauce, maple syrup, hot sauce, and ginger paste. Add mixture to vegetables and stir-fry for 2 to 3 minutes.
3. Turn heat off and dish salad. Drizzle with remaining avocado oil and garnish with sesame seeds.
4. Serve with grilled tofu.

Nutrition: calories 290, fat 1, carbs 8, protein 1

97. Broccoli, Kelp, and Feta Salad

Preparation Time: 15 Minutes

Cooking Time: 0

Servings: 4

Ingredients:

- 2 tbsp. olive oil
- 1 tbsp. white wine vinegar
- 2 tbsp. chia seeds
- Salt and freshly ground black pepper to taste
- 2 cups broccoli slaw
- 1 cup chopped kelp, thoroughly washed, and steamed
- 1/3 cup chopped pecans
- 1/3 cup pumpkin seeds
- 1/3 cup blueberries
- 2/3 cup ricotta cheese

Directions:

1. In a small bowl, whisk olive oil, white wine vinegar, chia seeds, salt, and black pepper. Set aside.
2. In a large salad bowl, combine the broccoli slaw, kelp, pecans, pumpkin seeds, blueberries, and ricotta cheese.
3. Drizzle dressing on top, toss, and serve.

Nutrition: calories 390, fat 3, carbs 8, protein 8

98. Roasted Asparagus with Feta Cheese Salad

Preparation Time: 10 minutes

Cooking Time: 20 minutes

Serving: 4

Ingredients:

- 1 lb. asparagus, trimmed and halved
- 2 tbsp. olive oil
- ½ tsp. dried basil
- ½ tsp. dried oregano
- Salt and freshly ground black pepper to taste
- ½ tsp. hemp seeds
- 1 tbsp. maple (sugar-free) syrup

- ½ cup arugula
- 4 tbsp. crumbled feta cheese
- 2 tbsp. hazelnuts
- 1 lemon, cut into wedges

Directions:

1. Preheat oven to 3500F.
2. Pour asparagus on a baking tray, drizzle with olive oil, basil, oregano, salt, black pepper, and hemp seeds. Mix with your hands and roast in the oven for 15 minutes.
3. Remove, drizzle with maple syrup, and continue cooking until slightly charred for 5 minutes.
4. Spread arugula in a salad bowl and top with asparagus. Scatter with feta cheese, hazelnuts, and serve with lemon wedges.

Nutrition: calories 140, fat 3, carbs 18, protein 4

99. Fresh Veggie Salad

Preparation Time: 20 Minutes

Cooking Time: 0

Servings: 8

Ingredients:

For Dressing:

- 5 tablespoons olive oil
- 3 tablespoons fresh lemon juice
- 2 tablespoons fresh mint leaves, chopped finely
- 1 teaspoon Erythritol
- Salt and freshly ground black pepper, to taste

For Salad:

- 2 cups cucumbers, peeled and sliced
- 2 cups tomatoes, sliced
- 1 cup black olives
- 6 cups lettuce

- 1 cup mozzarella cheese, cubed

Directions:

1. For the dressing: in a bowl, add all ingredients and beat until well combined.
2. Cover and refrigerate to chill for about 1 hour.
3. For the salad: in a large serving bowl, add all ingredients and mix.
4. Pour dressing over salad and toss to coat well.
5. Serve immediately.

Nutrition: calories 321, fat 1, carbs 8, protein 1

100. Strawberry Salad

Preparation Time: 15 Minutes

Cooking Time: 0

Servings: 4

Ingredients:

- 6 cups fresh baby greens
- 2 cups fresh strawberries, hulled and sliced
- 1 tablespoon fresh mint leaves
- ¼ cup olive oil
- 2 tablespoons fresh lemon juice
- ¼ teaspoon liquid stevia
- 1/8 teaspoon paprika
- 1/8 teaspoon garlic powder
- Salt, to taste

Directions:

1. For the salad: in a large serving bowl, add greens, strawberries, and mint and mix.
2. For the dressing: in a bowl, add remaining ingredients and beat until well combined.
3. Pour dressing over salad and toss to coat well.
4. Serve immediately.

Nutrition: calories 141, fat 2, carbs 18, protein 9

101. Tex Mex Black Bean and Avocado Salad

Preparation Time: 15 Minutes

Cooking Time: 0

Servings: 2

Ingredients:

- 14 oz. black beans, drained and rinsed
- 3 jars roasted red peppers, chopped
- 1 avocado, chopped
- ½ onion, chopped
- 1 red chili, chopped
- 1 lime, plus wedges to serve
- Olive oil
- 1 teaspoon cumin seeds
- 2 handfuls rocket
- 2 pitta breads, warmed

Directions:

1. Combine beans, peppers, avocado, onion, and chili in a large mixing bowl.
2. Add lime juice, cumin seeds, and mix well.
3. Serve the rocket on two plates with warm pittas and divide the bean mixture.

Nutrition: calories 120, fat 3, carbs 8, protein 5

102. Sweet Potato Salad

Preparation: 10 Minutes

Cooking Time: 30 Minutes

Servings: 4

Ingredients:

- 2 sweet potatoes, peeled and cubed
- 1 tablespoon olive oil
- ½ teaspoon each of paprika, oregano, and cayenne pepper
- 1 shallot, diced

- 2 spring onions, chopped
- 1 small bunch chives, chopped
- 3 tablespoons red wine vinegar
- 2 teaspoons olive oil
- 1 tablespoon pure maple syrup
- Salt and pepper

Directions:

1. Preheat the oven to 300F and prepare a baking sheet by lining it with parchment paper.
2. Place sweet potatoes on the baking sheet.
3. Drizzle some olive oil and spices, toss well, and bake for 30 minutes.
4. In a separate bowl, mix shallots, scallions, chives, vinegar, olive oil, and maple syrup.
5. Add baked sweet potatoes to the dressing.

Nutrition: calories 169, fat 1, carbs 5, protein 1

103. Lentil Salad with Spinach and Pomegranate

Preparation Time: 15 Minutes

Cooking Time: 0

Servings: 3

Ingredients

For the vegan lentil salad:

- 3 cups brown lentils, cooked
- 1 avocado, cut into slices
- 2-3 handfuls fresh spinach
- ½ cup walnuts, chopped
- 2 apples, chopped
- 1 pomegranate

For the tahini orange dressing:

- 3 tablespoons tahini
- 2 tablespoons olive oil

- 1 clove of garlic
- 6 tablespoons water
- 4 tablespoons orange juice
- 2 teaspoons orange zest
- Salt and pepper

Directions:

1. Prepare lentils according to package instructions.
2. Place pomegranate in a shallow bowl filled with water, cut in half, and take out seeds, remove fibers floating on the water.
3. Process all dressing ingredients in a food processor. Process until smooth and set aside.
4. Place salad ingredients in a large bowl and mix well.
5. Drizzle dressing over salad before serving.

Nutrition: calories 104, fat 3, carbs 18, protein 11

104. Broccoli Salad Curry Dressing

Preparation Time: 30 Minutes

Cooking Time: 0

Servings: 6

Ingredients:

- ½ cup plain, unsweetened vegan yogurt
- ¼ cup onion, chopped
- 2 heads broccoli florets, chopped
- 2 stalks celery, chopped
- ½ teaspoon curry powder
- ¼ teaspoon salt or to taste
- 2 tablespoons sunflower seeds

Directions:

1. Mix yogurt, curry powder, and salt.
2. Toss broccoli florets, celery onion, and sunflower seeds.
3. Drizzle the dressing on top and put the salad in the fridge for 30 minutes.

Nutrition: calories 167, fat 1, carbs 18, protein 1

105. Cherry Tomato Salad with Soy Chorizo

Preparation Time: 5 Minutes

Cooking Time: 5 Minutes

Servings: 4

Ingredients:

- 2 ½ tbsp. olive oil
- 4 soy chorizos, chopped
- 2 tsp. red wine vinegar
- 1 small red onion, finely chopped
- 2 ½ cups cherry tomatoes, halved
- 2 tbsp. chopped cilantro
- Salt and freshly ground black pepper to taste
- 3 tbsp. sliced black olives to garnish

Directions:

1. Heat half a tablespoon of olive oil in a skillet over a medium heat and fry soy chorizo until golden. Turn heat off.
2. In a salad bowl, whisk remaining olive oil and vinegar. Add onion, cilantro, tomatoes, and soy chorizo. Mix with dressing and season with salt and black pepper.
3. Garnish with olives and serve.

Nutrition: calories 130, fat 1, carbs 7, protein 1

106. Roasted Bell Pepper Salad with Olives

Preparation Time: 10 Minutes

Cooking Time: 20 Minutes

Servings: 4

Ingredients:

- 8 large red bell peppers, deseeded and cut in wedges
- ½ tsp. erythritol

- 2 ½ tbsp. olive oil
- 1/3 cup arugula
- 1 tbsp. mint leaves
- 1/3 cup pitted Kalamata olives
- 3 tbsp. chopped almonds
- ½ tbsp. balsamic vinegar
- Crumbled feta cheese for topping
- Toasted pine nuts for topping

Directions:

1. Preheat oven to 400 F.
2. Pour bell peppers on a roasting pan; season with erythritol and drizzle with half of the olive oil. Roast in oven until slightly charred, 20 minutes. Remove from the oven and set aside.
3. Arrange arugula in a salad bowl, scatter bell peppers on top, mint leaves, olives, almonds, and drizzle with balsamic vinegar and remaining olive oil. Season with salt and black pepper.
4. Toss, top with feta cheese and pine nuts, and serve.

Nutrition: calories 145, fat 1, carbs 8, protein 1

107. Tofu-Dulse-Walnut Salad

Preparation Time: 10 Minutes

Cooking Time: 15 Minutes

Servings: 4

Ingredients:

- 1 (7 oz.) block extra firm tofu
- 2 tbsp. olive oil
- 2 tbsp. butter
- 1 cup asparagus, trimmed and halved
- 1 cup green beans, trimmed
- 2 tbsp. chopped dulse
- Salt and freshly ground black pepper to taste
- ½ lemon, juiced

- 4 tbsp. chopped walnuts

Directions:

1. Place tofu in between two paper towels and allow soaking for 5 minutes. After, remove towels and chop into small cubes.
2. Heat olive oil in a skillet and fry tofu until golden, 10 minutes. Remove onto a paper towel-lined plate and set aside.
3. Melt butter in a skillet and sauté asparagus and green beans until softened, 5 minutes. Add dulse, season with salt and black pepper, and cook until softened. Mix in tofu and stir-fry for 5 minutes.
4. Plate, drizzle with lemon juice, and scatter walnuts on top.
5. Serve warm.

Nutrition: calories 178, fat 1, carbs 9, protein 1

108. Green Quinoa Salad

Preparation Time: 5 minutes

Cooking Time: 0 minutes

Serving: 4

Ingredients:

- 1 cup trimmed, cooked, and roughly chopped asparagus spears
- 1 cup roughly chopped radish florets
- 1/2 tsp. sea salt
- 2 tbsps. Coconut oil
- 2 tbsps. Freshly squeezed Seville orange juice
- 1/2 cup water
- 2 cups cooled cooked quinoa

Directions:

1. In a bowl, mix the radish and asparagus.
2. Add in the quinoa then stir.
3. Mix the water, coconut oil, salt, and Seville orange juice using a blender.
4. Blend until the ingredients emulsify.
5. Pour the mixture over the salad then stir to mix.
6. Keep the salad in the fridge for about 15 minutes to chill.

7. Serve cold.

Nutrition: calories 121, fat 1, carbs 11, protein 1

109. Salad Pop

Preparation Time: 5 minutes

Cooking Time: 0 minutes

Serving: 4

Ingredients:

- 1 yellow squash, sliced into pieces
- 1 zucchini, sliced into pieces
- 1 cucumber, sliced into pieces
- 8 cauliflower florets
- 2 tbsps. Blue cheese dressing
- 8 steamed radish florets
- 8 cherry tomatoes

Directions:

1. Thread 1 zucchini slice onto a wooden skewer, followed by the 1 yellow squash slice, 1 cucumber, 1 cherry tomato, 1 radish floret, and 1 cauliflower floret.
2. Repeat the process with the remaining ingredients and vegetable pieces.
3. Drizzle with the blue cheese dressing.
4. Serve.

Nutrition: calories 143, fat 1, carbs 18, protein 7

110. Avocado Power Salad

Preparation Time: 10 minutes

Cooking Time: 0 minutes

Serving: 2

Ingredients:

- 1 cubed avocado
- 1 cup cooled cooked quinoa
- 1 tbsp. freshly squeezed Seville orange juice
- 1 tsp. sea salt
- 1 tbsp. onion powder
- 1 tbsp. onion powder
- 1/4 cup chopped cilantro
- 1 cup peeled and diced cucumber
- 1 cup halved cherry tomatoes
- 5oz. fresh and roughly chopped kale

Directions:

1. Mix all the ingredients.
2. Place the mixture in the fridge to chill for about 15 minutes
3. Serve.

Nutrition: calories 211, fat 2, carbs 18, protein 5

111. Wakame Salad

Preparation Time: 10 minutes

Cooking Time: 15 minutes

Serving: 2

Ingredients

- 2 cups of Wakame Stems
- 1 tablespoon of Sesame Seeds
- 2 tablespoons of diced Red Bell Pepper
- 1 teaspoon of Ginger
- 1 tablespoon of Agave Syrup
- 1 teaspoon of Onion Powder
- 1 tablespoon of Sesame Oil
- 1 tablespoon of Key Lime juice
- Spring Water for soaking

Direction:

1. Put wakame stems in a medium bowl and cover them with spring water.
2. Soak wakame stems for 8 to 10 minutes until soft then drain the water.
3. In a separate bowl, combine agave syrup, onion powder, sesame oil, ginger, and key lime juice and whisk them thoroughly.
4. Place diced bell pepper and soaked wakame on a plate. Pour dressing over the salad.
5. Sprinkle sesame seeds on top.
6. Enjoy your wakame salad!

Nutrition: calories 190, fat 1, carbs 18, protein 1

112. Healthy Salad

Preparation Time: 10 minutes

Cooking Time: 54 minutes

Serving: 2

Ingredients

- 2 cups of torn Watercress
- 1/2 of sliced Cucumber
- 1 tablespoon of Key Lime Juice
- 2 tablespoons of Olive Oil
- Pure Sea Salt, to taste
- Cayenne Powder, to taste

Direction:

1. Pour key lime juice and olive oil into a salad bowl. Mix them well to combine.
2. Slice the cucumber and add to the bowl.
3. Tear watercress and add to the bowl.
4. Sprinkle cayenne powder and pure sea salt on top according to your liking.
5. Mix thoroughly.
6. Enjoy your quick detox salad!

Nutrition: calories 265, fat 1, carbs 9, protein 1

Chapter 9

SPECIAL INGREDIENTS

113. Homemade Hemp Seed Milk

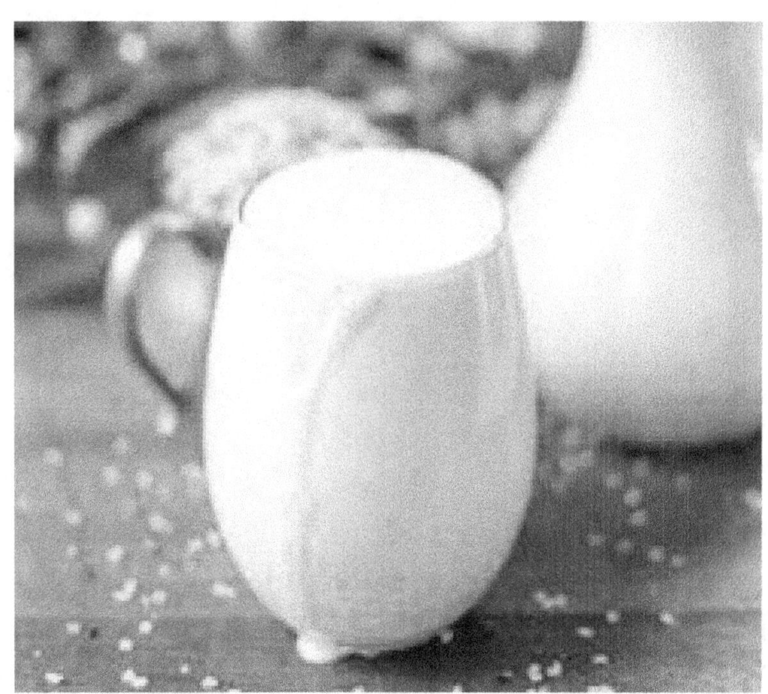

Preparation Time: 15 minutes

Cooking Time: 2 hours

Servings: 2

Ingredients:

- 2 tablespoons of hemp seeds
- 2 tablespoons of agave syrup

- 1/8 teaspoon of pure sea salt
- 2 cups of spring water
- Fruits (optional)*

Directions:

1. Place all ingredients, except fruits, into the blender.
2. Blend them for two minutes.
3. Add fruits and repeatedly blend for 30 to 50 seconds.
4. Leave milk in a refrigerator until cold.
5. Enjoy your homemade hemp seed milk!

Nutrition: calories 211, fat 1, carbs 8, protein 1

114. Italian Infused Oil

Preparation Time: 5 minutes

Cooking Time: 24 hours

Servings: 1

Ingredients:

- 1 teaspoon of oregano
- 1 teaspoon of basil
- 1 pinch of pure sea salt
- 3/4 cup of grapeseed oil

Directions:

1. Fill a glass jar with a lid or a squeeze bottle with grapeseed oil.
2. Mix seasoning together and add them to the jar/bottle.
3. Shake it and let the oil infuse for at least 24 hours.
4. Add it to a dish and enjoy your Italian infused oil!

Nutrition: calories 120, fat 1, carbs 10, protein 1

115. Garlic Infused Oil

Preparation Time: 5 minutes

Cooking Time: 24 hours

Servings: 1

Ingredients:

- 1/2 teaspoon of dill
- 1/2 teaspoon of ginger powder
- 1 tablespoon of onion powder
- 1/2 teaspoon of pure sea salt
- 3/4 cup of grapeseed oil

Directions:

1. Fill a glass jar with a lid or a squeeze bottle with Grape Seed Oil.
2. Add the seasonings to the jar/bottle.
3. Shake it and let the oil infuse for at least 24 hours.
4. Add it to a dish and enjoy your "Garlic" Infused Oil!

Nutrition: calories 130, fat 4, carbs 19, protein 2

116. Papaya Seed Mango Dressing

Preparation Time: 5 minutes

Cooking Time: 10 minutes

Servings: 2

Ingredients:

- 1 cup of chopped mango
- 1 teaspoon of ground papaya seeds
- 1 teaspoon of basil
- 1 teaspoon of onion powder
- 1 teaspoon of agave syrup
- 2 tablespoons of lime juice
- 1/4 cup of grapeseed oil
- 1/4 teaspoon of pure sea salt

Directions:

1. Prepare and place all ingredients into the blender.
2. Blend for one minute until smooth.
3. Add it to a salad and enjoy your papaya seed mango dressing!

Nutrition: calories 320, fat 12, carbs 18, protein 1

117. Tomato Ginger Dressing

Preparation Time: 5 minutes

Cooking Time: 10 minutes

Servings: 2

Ingredients:

- 2 chopped plum tomatoes
- 1 teaspoon of minced ginger*
- 1 tablespoon of agave syrup
- 2 tablespoons of chopped onion
- 2 tablespoons of sesame seeds
- 1 tablespoon of lime juice

Directions:

1. Prepare and place all ingredients into the blender.
2. Blend for one minute until smooth.
3. Add it to a salad and enjoy your tomato ginger dressing!

Nutrition: calories 1, fat 3, carbs 18, protein 11

118. Dill Cucumber Dressing

Preparation Time: 5 minutes

Cooking Time: 10 minutes

Servings: 2

Ingredients:

- 1 teaspoon of fresh dill*
- 1 cup of quartered cucumbers
- 1/2 teaspoon of onion powder
- 2 teaspoons of agave syrup
- 1 tablespoon of lime juice
- 1/4 cup of Avocado oil

Directions:

1. Prepare and place all ingredients into the blender.
2. Blend for one minute until smooth.
3. Add it to a salad and enjoy your dill cucumber dressing!

Nutrition: calories 111, fat 3, carbs 18, protein 11

119. Homemade Walnut Milk

Preparation Time: 15 minutes

Cooking Time: Minimum 8 hours

Servings: 4 cups

Ingredients:

- 1 cup of raw walnuts
- 1/8 teaspoon of pure sea salt
- 3 cups of spring water + extra for soaking

Directions:

1. Put raw walnuts in a small pot and cover them with three inches of water.
2. Soak the walnuts for at least eight hours.
3. Drain and rinse the walnuts with cold water.
4. Add the soaked walnuts, pure sea salt, and three cups of spring water to a blender.
5. Mix well until smooth.
6. Strain it if you need to.
7. Enjoy your homemade walnut milk!

Nutrition: calories 118, fat 111, carbs 18, protein 1

120. Aquafaba

Preparation Time: 15 minutes

Cooking Time: 2 Hours 30 Minutes

Servings: 2-4 Cups

Ingredients:

- 1 bag of garbanzo beans
- 1 teaspoon of pure sea salt
- 6 cups of spring water + extra for soaking

Directions:

1. Place garbanzo beans in a large pot, add spring water and pure sea salt. Bring to a rolling boil.
2. Remove from the heat and leave to soak kindly for 30 to 40 minutes.
3. Strain garbanzo beans and add 6 cups of spring water.
4. Boil for 1 hour and 30 minutes on medium heat.
5. Strain the garbanzo beans. This strained water is Aquafaba.
6. Pour Aquafaba into a glass jar with a lid and place it into the refrigerator.
7. After cooling, Aquafaba becomes thicker. If it is too liquid, repeatedly boil for 10-20 minutes.

Nutrition: calories 234, fat 10, carbs 9, protein 11

121. Potato and Zucchini Casserole

Preparation Time: 10 Minutes

Cooking Time: 1 hour

Servings: 6

Ingredients:

- ¾ cup nutritional yeast
- ¾ cup diced green or red bell pepper (about one small bell pepper)
- ¾ cup diced red, white, or yellow onion (about one small onion)
- ½ cup dry breadcrumbs
- ¼ cup olive oil (optional)
- 1½ teaspoons minced garlic (about three small cloves)
- Pepper, to taste
- Sea salt, to taste (optional)

Directions:

1. Preheat the oven to 400⁰F.
2. Mix all the ingredients.
3. Place the mixture in a large cooking pot dish.
4. Bake in a preheated oven for 1 hour until heated through, stirring once halfway through.
5. Take off from the oven and allow to cool for 5 minutes before serving.

Nutrition: calories 321, fat 10, carbs 38, protein 14

122. Broccoli Casserole with Beans and Walnuts

Preparation Time: 10 Minutes

Cooking Time: 35-40 Minutes

Servings: 4

Ingredients:

- ¾ cup vegetable broth
- Two broccoli heads, crowns, and stalks finely chopped
- One teaspoon salt (optional)
- 2 cups cooked pinto or navy beans
- 1 to 2 tablespoons brown rice flour or arrowroot flour
- 1 cup chopped walnuts

Directions:

1. Preheat the oven to 400⁰F (205⁰C).
2. Warm the vegetable broth in a large ovenproof pot over medium heat.
3. Add the broccoli and season with salt, if desired, then cook for 6 to 8 minutes, stirring occasionally, or until the broccoli is light green.
4. Add the pinto beans and brown rice flour to the skillet and stir well. Sauté for another 5 to 7 minutes, or until the liquid thickens slightly. Scatter the top with the walnuts.
5. Transfer the pot to the oven. Bake it until the walnuts are toasted, 20 to 25 minutes.
6. Let the casserole cool for 8 to 10 minutes in the pot before serving.

Nutrition: calories 419, fat 2, carbs 18, protein 11

123. Pistachio Crusted Tofu

Preparation Time: 10 Minutes

Cooking Time: 20 Minutes

Servings: 8

Ingredients:

- ½ cup roasted, shelled pistachios
- ¼ cup whole wheat breadcrumbs
- One garlic clove, minced
- One shallot, minced
- ½ teaspoon dried tarragon
- One teaspoon grated lemon zest
- Sea salt, to taste (optional)
- Black pepper, to taste
- One tablespoon Dijon mustard
- One tablespoon lemon juice

Directions:

1. Warm up the oven to 400°F (205°C). Line a baking sheet with parchment paper.
2. Then place the pistachios in a food processor until they are about the size of the breadcrumbs. Mix the pistachios, breadcrumbs, garlic, shallot, tarragon, and lemon zest in a shallow dish. Sprinkle with salt (if desired) and pepper. Set aside.
3. Sprinkle the tofu with salt (if desired) and pepper. Mix the mustard and lemon juice in a small bowl and stir well.
4. Brush all over the tofu with the mustard mixture, then coat each slice with the pistachio mixture.
5. Arrange the tofu on the baking sheet. Scatter any remaining pistachio mixture over the slices.
6. Bake in the warmed oven for about 18 to 20 minutes, or until the tofu is browned and crispy.
7. Serve hot.

Nutrition: calories 159, fat 9, carbs 48, protein 10

124. Instant Savory Gigante Beans

Preparation Time: 10-30 Minutes

Cooking Time: 55 Minutes

Servings: 6

Ingredients:

- 1 lb. Gigante Beans soaked overnight
- 1/2 cup olive oil
- One onion sliced
- Two cloves garlic crushed or minced
- One red bell pepper (cut into 1/3-inch pieces)
- Two carrots, sliced
- 1/2 tsp salt and ground black pepper
- Two tomatoes peeled, grated
- 1 Tbsp celery (chopped)
- 1 tbsp tomato paste (or ketchup)
- 3/4 tsp sweet paprika
- 1 tsp oregano
- 1 cup vegetable broth

Directions:

1. Soak Gigante beans overnight.
2. Press the SAUTÉ button on your Instant Pot and heat the oil.
3. Sauté onion, garlic, sweet pepper, carrots with a pinch of salt for 3 - 4 minutes; stir occasionally.
4. Add rinsed Gigante beans into your Instant Pot along with all remaining ingredients and stir well.
5. Latch lid into place and set on the MANUAL setting for 25 minutes.
6. When the beep sounds, quick release the pressure by pressing Cancel and twisting the steam handle to the Venting position.
7. Taste and adjust seasonings to taste.
8. Serve warm or cold.
9. Keep refrigerated.

Nutrition: calories 232, fat 18, carbs 21, protein 9

125. Instant Turmeric Risotto

Preparation Time: 10-30 Minutes

Cooking Time: 40 Minutes

Servings: 4

Ingredients:

- 4 Tbsp olive oil
- 1 cup onion
- 1 tsp minced garlic
- 2 cups long-grain rice
- 3 cups vegetable broth
- 1/2 tsp paprika (smoked)
- 1/2 tsp turmeric
- 1/2 tsp nutmeg
- 2 Tbsp fresh basil leaves chopped
- Salt and ground black pepper to taste

Directions:

1. Press the SAUTÉ button on your Instant Pot and heat oil.
2. Sauté the onion and garlic with a pinch of salt until softened.
3. Add the rice and all leftover ingredients and stir well.
4. Lock the lid into place and set on and select the RICE button for 10 minutes.
5. Press Cancel when the timer beeps and carefully flip the Quick Release valve to let the pressure out.
6. Taste and adjust seasonings to taste.
7. Serve.

Nutrition: calories 154, fat 10, carbs 18, protein 9

126. Nettle Soup with Rice

Preparation Time: 10-30 Minutes

Cooking Time: 40 Minutes

Servings: 5

Ingredients:

- 3 Tbsp of olive oil
- Two onions finely chopped
- Two cloves garlic finely chopped
- Salt and freshly ground black pepper
- Four medium potatoes cut into cubes
- 1 cup of rice
- 1 Tbsp arrowroot
- 2 cups vegetable broth
- 2 cups of water
- One bunch of young nettle leaves packed
- 1/2 cup fresh parsley finely chopped
- 1 tsp cumin

Directions:

1. Heat olive oil in a large pot.
2. Sauté onion and garlic with a pinch of salt until softened.
3. Add potato, rice, and arrowroot; sauté for 2 to 3 minutes.
4. Pour broth and water, stir well, cover and cook over medium heat for about 20 minutes.
5. Cook for about 30 to 45 minutes.
6. Add young nettle leaves, parsley, and cumin; stir and cook for 5 to 7 minutes.
7. Move the soup to a blender and blend until combined well.
8. Taste and adjust salt and pepper.
9. Serve hot.

Nutrition: calories 419, fat 1, carbs 18, protein 11

127. Okra with Grated Tomatoes

Preparation Time: 10-30 Minutes

Cooking Time: 3 Hours and 10 Minutes

Servings: 4

Ingredients:

- 2 lbs. fresh okra cleaned
- Two onions finely chopped
- Two cloves garlic finely sliced
- Two carrots sliced
- Two ripe tomatoes grated
- 1 cup of water
- 4 Tbsp olive oil
- Salt and ground black pepper
- 1 tbsp fresh parsley finely chopped

Directions:

1. Add okra in your Crock-Pot: sprinkle with a pinch of salt and pepper.
2. Add in chopped onion, garlic, carrots, and grated tomatoes; stir well.
3. Pour water and oil, season with the salt, pepper, and give a good stir.
4. Cover and cook on LOW for 2-4 hours or until tender.
5. Open the lid and add fresh parsley; stir.
6. Taste and adjust salt and pepper.
7. Serve hot.

Nutrition: calories 223, fat 13, carbs 9, protein 14

128. Oven-Baked Smoked Lentil Burgers

Preparation Time: 10-30 Minutes

Cooking Time: 1 Hour and 20 Minutes

Servings: 6

Ingredients:

- 1 1/2 cups dried lentils
- 3 cups of water
- Salt and ground black pepper to taste
- 2 Tbsp olive oil
- One onion finely diced
- Two cloves minced garlic
- 1 cup button mushrooms sliced
- 2 Tbsp tomato paste
- 1/2 tsp fresh basil finely chopped
- 1 cup chopped almonds
- 3 tsp balsamic vinegar
- 3 Tbsp coconut amino
- 1 tsp liquid smoke
- 3/4 cup silken tofu soft
- 3/4 cup corn starch

Directions:

1. Cook lentils in salted water until tender or for about 30-35 minutes; rinse, drain, and set aside.
2. Heat oil in a frying skillet and sauté onion, garlic, and mushrooms for 4 to 5 minutes; stir occasionally.
3. Stir in the tomato paste, salt, basil, salt, and black pepper; cook for 2 to 3 minutes.
4. Stir in almonds, vinegar, coconut amino, liquid smoke, and lentils.
5. Remove from heat and stir in blended tofu and corn starch.
6. Keep stirring until all ingredients combined well.
7. Form mixture into patties and refrigerate for an hour.
8. Preheat oven to 350 F.
9. Line a baking dish with parchment paper and arrange patties on the pan.
10. Bake for 20 to 25 minutes.
11. Serve hot with buns, green salad, tomato sauce, etc.

Nutrition: calories 169, fat 1, carbs 11, protein 8

129. Powerful Spinach and Mustard Leaves Puree

Preparation Time: 10-30 Minutes

Cooking Time: 50 Minutes

Servings: 4

Ingredients:

- 2 Tbsp almond butter
- One onion finely diced
- 2 Tbsp minced garlic
- 1 tsp salt and black pepper (or to taste)
- 1 lb. mustard leaves cleaned rinsed
- 1 lb. frozen spinach thawed
- 1 tsp coriander
- 1 tsp ground cumin
- 1/2 cup almond milk

Directions:

1. Press the SAUTÉ button on your Instant Pot and heat the almond butter.
2. Sauté onion, garlic, and a pinch of salt for 2-3 minutes; stir occasionally.
3. Add spinach and the mustard greens and stir for a minute or two.
4. Season with the salt and pepper, coriander, and cumin; give a good stir.
5. Lock lid into place and set on the MANUAL setting for 15 minutes.
6. Use Quick Release - turn the valve from sealing to venting to release the pressure.
7. Move mixture to a blender, add almond milk, and blend until smooth.
8. Taste and adjust seasonings.
9. Serve.

Nutrition: calories 180, fat 1, carbs 18, protein 10

Chapter 10

VEGETABLE

130. Power Pesto Zoodles

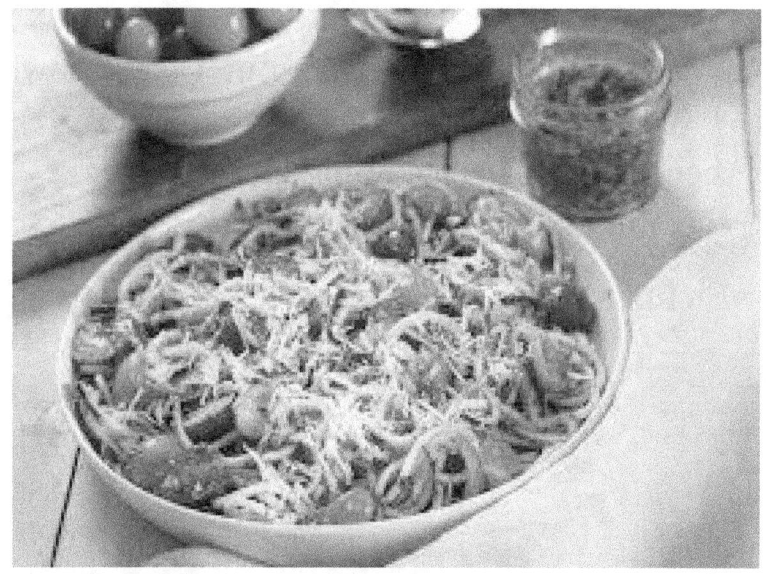

Preparation Time: 10 minutes

Cooking time: 5 minutes

Servings: 2

Ingredients:

- 2 zucchinis
- 1 avocado, peeled, pitted
- ½ cup cherry tomatoes
- 2 tablespoons walnuts

- ½ of key lime, juiced

Extra:

- ¼ teaspoon salt
- 1/8 teaspoon cayenne pepper
- 2 teaspoons grapeseed oil
- 2 tablespoons olive oil

Directions

1. Prepare the zucchini noodles and for this, cut them into thin strips by using a vegetable peeler or use a spiralizer.
2. Then take a medium skillet pan, add oil in it and when hot, add zucchini noodles in it and then cook for 3 to 5 minutes until tender-crisp.
3. Meanwhile, place the remaining ingredients in a food processor and then pulse until the creamy paste comes together.
4. When zucchini noodles have sautéed, drain and place them in a large bowl and add the blended sauce in it.
5. Add 2 tablespoons of water and then toss until well combined.
6. Garnish the zoodles with grated coconut and then serve.

Nutrition: calories 220, fat 11, carbs 18, protein 19

131. Mushroom Gravy

Preparation Time: 5 minutes

Cooking time: 12 minutes

Servings: 2

Ingredients:

- ¾ tablespoon spelt flour
- ¼ of onion, peeled, diced
- 4 ounces sliced mushrooms
- ½ cup walnut milk, homemade
- 1 tablespoon chopped walnuts

Extra:

- ¼ teaspoon salt
- 1/8 teaspoon cayenne pepper
- ½ teaspoon dried thyme
- 1 tablespoon grapeseed oil
- ¼ cup vegetable broth, homemade

Directions:

1. Take a medium skillet pan, place it over medium heat, add oil, and when hot, add onion and mushrooms, season with 1/16 teaspoon each of salt and cayenne pepper, and then cook for 4 minutes until tender.
2. Stir in spelt flour until coated, cook for 1 minute, slowly whisk in milk and vegetable broth and then season with remaining salt and cayenne pepper.
3. Switch heat to low-level, cook for 5 to 7 minutes until the sauce has thickened slightly, and then stir in walnuts and thyme.
4. Serve straight away with spelt flour bread.

Nutrition: calories 312, fat 8, carbs 18, protein 10

132. Nori Burritos

Preparation Time: 10 minutes

Cooking time: 0 minutes

Servings: 2

Ingredients:

- 1 avocado, peeled, sliced
- 1 cucumber, deseeded, cut into round slices
- 1 zucchini, sliced
- 2 teaspoons sprouted hemp seeds
- 2 nori sheets

Extra:

- 1 tablespoon tahini butter
- 2 teaspoons sesame seeds

Directions:

1. Working on one nori sheet at a time, place it on a cutting board shiny-side-down and then arrange half of each avocado, cucumber and zucchini slices and tahini on it, leaving 1-inch wide spice to the right.
2. Then start folding the sheet over the fillings from the edge that is closest to you, cut into thick slices, and then sprinkle with 1 teaspoon of sesame seeds.
3. Repeat with the remaining nori sheet, and then serve.

Nutrition: calories 210, fat 1, carbs 20, protein 11

133. Zesty Citrus Salad

Preparation Time: 5 minutes

Cooking time: 0 minutes

Servings: 2

Ingredients:

- 4 slices of onion
- ½ of avocado, peeled, pitted, sliced
- 4 ounces arugula
- 1 orange, zested, peeled, sliced
- 1 teaspoon agave syrup

Extra:

- 1/8 teaspoon salt
- 1/8 teaspoon cayenne pepper
- 2 tablespoons key lime juice
- 2 tablespoons olive oil

Directions:

1. Distribute avocado, oranges, onion, and arugula between two plates.
2. Mix together oil, salt, cayenne pepper, agave syrup, and lime juice in a small bowl and then stir until mixed.
3. Drizzle the dressing over the salad and then serve.

Nutrition: calories 276, fat 3, carbs 18, protein 11

134. Zucchini Hummus Wrap

Preparation Time: 10 minutes

Cooking time: 8 minutes

Servings: 2

Ingredients:

- ½ cup iceberg lettuce
- 1 zucchini, sliced
- 2 cherry tomatoes, sliced
- 2 spelt flour tortillas
- 4 tablespoons homemade hummus

Extra:

- ¼ teaspoon salt
- 1/8 teaspoon cayenne pepper
- 1 tablespoon grapeseed oil

Directions:

1. Take a grill pan, grease it with oil and let it preheat over medium-high heat setting.
2. Meanwhile, place zucchini slices in a large bowl, sprinkle with salt and cayenne pepper, drizzle with oil and then toss until coated.
3. Arrange zucchini slices on the grill pan and then cook for 2 to 3 minutes per side until developed grill marks.
4. Assemble tortillas and for this, heat the tortilla on the grill pan until warm and develop grill marks and spread 2 tablespoons of hummus over each tortilla.
5. Distribute grilled zucchini slices over the tortillas, top with lettuce and tomato slices, and then wrap tightly.
6. Serve straight away.

Nutrition: calories 132, fat 1, carbs 18, protein 10

135. Basil and Avocado Salad

Preparation Time: 10 minutes

Cooking time: 0 minutes

Servings: 2

Ingredients:

- ½ cup avocado, peeled, pitted, chopped
- ½ cup basil leaves
- ½ cup cherry tomatoes
- 2 cups cooked spelt noodles

Extra:

- 1 teaspoon agave syrup
- 1 tablespoon key lime juice
- 2 tablespoons olive oil

Directions:

1. Take a large bowl, place pasta in it, add tomato, avocado, and basil in it and then stir until mixed.
2. Take a small bowl, add agave syrup and salt in it, pour in lime juice and olive oil, and then whisk until combined.
3. Pour lime juice mixture over pasta, toss until combined, and then serve.

Nutrition: calories 188, fat 10, carbs 9, protein 22

136. Vegan Portobello Burgers

Preparation Time: 10 minutes

Cooking time: 20 minutes

Servings: 2

Ingredients:

- 2 Portobello mushroom caps
- ½ of avocado, sliced
- 1 cup purslane
- 2 teaspoons dried basil

- 2 tablespoons olive oil

Extra:

- ¼ teaspoon salt
- 1 teaspoon dried oregano
- ½ teaspoon cayenne pepper

Directions:

1. Switch on the oven, then set it to 425 degrees F and let it preheat.
2. Prepare the marinade and for this, take a small bowl, pour in oil, add cayenne pepper, onion powder, oregano, and basil and then stir until mixed.
3. Take a cookie sheet, line it with a foil, brush with oil, place mushroom caps on it, evenly pour the marinade over mushroom caps and then let them marinate for 10 minutes.
4. Then bake the mushroom caps for 20 minutes, flipping halfway, until tender and cooked.
5. When done, place mushroom caps on two plates, top the caps with avocado and purslane evenly and then serve.

Nutrition: calories 132, fat 13, carbs 18, protein 28

137. Grilled Romaine Lettuce Salad

Preparation Time: 10 minutes

Cooking time: 10 minutes

Servings: 2

Ingredients:

- 2 small heads of romaine lettuce, cut in half
- 1 tablespoon chopped basil
- 1 tablespoon chopped red onion
- ¼ teaspoon onion powder
- ½ tablespoon agave syrup

Extra:

- ½ teaspoon salt
- ¼ teaspoon cayenne pepper

- 2 tablespoons olive oil
- 1 tablespoon key lime juice

Directions:

1. Take a large skillet pan, place it over medium heat and when warmed, arrange lettuce heads in it, cut-side down, and then cook for 4 to 5 minutes per side until golden brown on both sides.
2. When done, transfer lettuce heads to a plate and then let them cool for 5 minutes.
3. Meanwhile, prepare the dressing and for this, place remaining ingredients in a small bowl and then stir until combined.
4. Drizzle the dressing over lettuce heads and then serve.

Nutrition: calories 190, fat 18, carbs 18, protein 32

138. Vegetable Fajitas

Preparation Time: 10 minutes

Cooking time: 8 minutes

Servings: 2

Ingredients:

- 2 Portobello mushroom caps, 1/3-inch sliced
- ¾ of red bell pepper, sliced
- ½ of onion, peeled, sliced
- ½ of key lime, juiced
- 2 spelt flour tortillas

Extra:

- 1/3 teaspoon salt
- ¼ teaspoon cayenne pepper
- ¼ teaspoon onion powder
- 1 tablespoon grapeseed oil

Directions

1. Take a medium skillet pan, place it over medium heat, add oil, and when hot, add onion and red pepper, and then cook for 2 minutes until tender-crisp.

2. Add mushrooms slices, sprinkle with all the seasoning, stir until mixed, and then cook for 5 minutes until vegetables turn soft.
3. Heat the tortilla until warm, distribute vegetables in their center, drizzle with lime juice, and then roll tightly.
4. Serve straight away.

Nutrition: calories 220, fat 23, carbs 12, protein 28

139. Appetizing Baked Apple

Preparation Time: 10 minutes

Cooking time: 55 minutes

Servings: 2

Ingredients:

- 4 apples, large, cored, sliced
- 1/8 teaspoon ground cloves
- 3 tablespoons agave syrup
- 1 tablespoon chopped walnuts

Directions

1. Switch on the oven, then set it to 350 degrees F and let it preheat.
2. Meanwhile, take a large bowl, place apple slices in it, drizzle with agave syrup and then toss until evenly coated.
3. Take a small bowl, place nuts in it, add cloves, and then stir until mixed.
4. Sprinkle nuts mixture over the apple and let it rest for 5 minutes or more until apples start releasing their juices.
5. Take a medium casserole dish, arrange apple slices on it, and then bake for 15 minutes.
6. Cover the casserole dish with foil and then continue baking for 40 minutes until bubbly.
7. Let apples cool for 10 minutes and then serve.

Nutrition: calories 184, fat 20, carbs 18, protein 26

140. Classic Banana Fries

Preparation Time: 5 minutes

Cooking time: 10 minutes

Servings: 2

Ingredients:

- 4 baby burro bananas, peeled, cut into squares
- ¼ teaspoon salt
- ½ of a medium onion, peeled, chopped
- ½ of medium green bell pepper, cored, chopped
- 2 teaspoons grapeseed oil

Extra:

- ¼ teaspoon cayenne pepper

Directions

1. Take a medium skillet pan, place it over medium-low heat, add oil, and when hot, add burro banana pieces, and then cook for 3 minutes or until beginning to brown.
2. Then turn the burro banana pieces, add remaining ingredients, stir until mixed, and then continue cooking for 5 to 7 minutes until onions have caramelized.
3. Serve straight away.

Nutrition: calories 188, fat 18, carbs 10, protein 32

141. Zoodles with Basil & Avocado Sauce

Preparation Time: 10 minutes

Cooking time: 0 minutes

Servings: 2

Ingredients:

- 2 zucchinis, spiralized into noodles
- 2 avocados, peeled, pitted
- ½ cup walnuts

- 2 cups basil leaves
- 24 cherry tomatoes, sliced

Extra:

- 1/3 teaspoon salt
- 4 tablespoons key lime juice
- ½ cup spring water

Directions:

1. Prepare the sauce and for this, place all the ingredients except for zucchini noodles and tomatoes in a food processor and then pulse until smooth.
2. Take a large bowl, place zucchini noodles in it, add tomato slices, pour in the prepared sauce, and then toss until coated.
3. Serve straight away.

Nutrition: calories 188, fat 21, carbs 10, protein 22

142. Butternut Squash and Apple Burger

Preparation Time: 10 minutes

Cooking time: 1 hour

Servings: 2

Ingredients:

- ¾ cup diced butternut squash
- ½ cup diced apples
- 1 cup cooked wild rice
- ¼ cup chopped shallots
- ½ tablespoon thyme

Extra:

- ¼ teaspoon sea salt, divided
- 1 tablespoon pumpkin seeds, unsalted
- 1 tablespoon grapeseed oil
- 2 spelt burgers, halved, toasted

Directions

1. Switch on the oven, then set it to 400 degrees F and let it preheat.
2. Meanwhile, take a cookie sheet, line it with parchment sheet, spread squash pieces on it and then sprinkle with 1/8 teaspoon salt.
3. Bake the squash for 15 minutes, then add shallots and apple, sprinkle with remaining salt, and then bake for 20 to 30 minutes until cooked.
4. When done, let the vegetable mixture cool for 15 minutes, transfer it into a food processor, add thyme and then pulse until a chunky mixture comes together.
5. Add pumpkin seeds and cooked wild rice, pulse until combined, and then tip the mixture in a bowl.
6. Taste the mixture to adjust and then shape it into two patties.
7. Take a skillet pan, place it over medium heat, add oil and when hot, place patties in it and then cook for 5 to 7 minutes per side until browned.
8. Sandwich patties in burger buns and then serve.

Nutrition: calories 210, fat 13, carbs 18, protein 21

143. Kale and Avocado Dish

Preparation Time: 5 minutes

Cooking time: 0 minutes

Servings: 2

Ingredients

- 1 bundle of kale, cut into thin strips
- 1 small white onion, peeled, chopped
- 12 cherry tomatoes, chopped
- 1 tablespoon salt
- 1 avocado, peeled, pitted, sliced

Directions

1. Take a large bowl, place kale strips in it, sprinkle with salt, and then massage for 2 minutes.
2. Cover the bowl with a plastic wrap or its lid, let it rest for a minimum of 30 minutes, and then stir in onion and tomatoes until well combined.

3. Let the salad sit for 5 minutes, add avocado slices, and then serve.

Nutrition: calories 110, fat 19, carbs 7, protein 21

<u>Chapter 11</u>

DINNER RECIPES

144. Roasted Sweet Potatoes

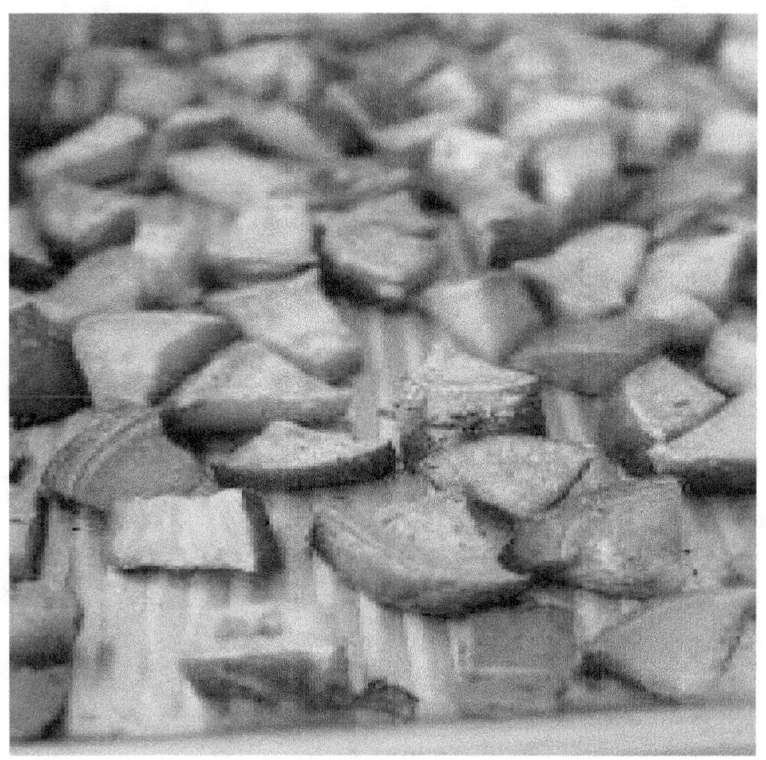

Preparation time: 10 minutes

Cooking time: 45 minutes

Servings: 4

Ingredients:

- 2 sweet potatoes, peeled and cubed
- 2½ tablespoons avocado oil
- A pinch of salt and black pepper
- 1 garlic clove, minced
- Juice of 1 lime
- 4 tablespoons water

Directions:

1. Spread the potatoes on a lined baking sheet and combine with the rest of the ingredients.
2. Cook at 400 degrees F for 45 minutes and serve for lunch.

Nutrition: calories 222, fat 6, carbs 15, protein 7

145. Lemony Carrot Soup

Preparation time: 10 minutes

Cooking time: 40 minutes

Servings: 4

Ingredients:

- 2 cups carrots, sliced
- 1 tablespoon olive oil
- 1 yellow onion, chopped
- 1½ cups kale, chopped
- 1 cup plum tomatoes, cubed
- 3 garlic cloves, minced
- A pinch of salt and black pepper
- 4 teaspoons fresh grated ginger
- 4 cups water
- 1 teaspoon sweet paprika
- 2 teaspoons ground turmeric
- Juice of 1 lemon
- Zest of ½ lemon, grated

Directions:

1. Heat up a pot with the oil over medium heat, add the onion and garlic, and cook for 5 minutes.
2. Add the carrots and the other ingredients, stir and simmer for 35 minutes more.
3. Divide into bowls and serve.

Nutrition: calories 271, fat 8, carbs 8,3, protein 8

146. Burrito Bowls

Preparation time: 10 minutes

Cooking time: 0 minutes

Servings: 1

Ingredients:

- ¼ cup spinach leaves, torn
- 1 tablespoon chives, chopped
- 1 tablespoon chopped red bell pepper
- 1 teaspoon olive oil
- 3 cherry tomatoes, halved
- 1 tablespoon chopped parsley
- 1 red cabbage, shredded
- Juice of 1 lime

Directions:

1. In a bowl, mix the spinach with the chives and the other ingredients, toss, and serve for lunch.

Nutrition: calories 207, fat 3.8, carbs 6, protein 4.4

147. Mixed Beans Bowls

Preparation time: 10 minutes

Cooking time: 40 minutes

Servings: 4

Ingredients:

- 1 cup pinto beans, rinsed
- 1 cup red beans, rinsed
- 1 cup white beans, rinsed
- 1 cup soybeans, rinsed
- 1 yellow onions, chopped
- 1 tablespoon avocado oil
- 1 cup cherry tomatoes, halved
- 1 cup baby spinach
- 1 small jalapeno pepper, minced
- 2 teaspoons lime juice
- Zest of 1 lime, grated
- Salt and black pepper to the taste
- 1 teaspoon turmeric powder

Directions:

1. Heat up a pan with the oil over medium heat, add the onion, jalapeno and turmeric and cook for 5 minutes.
2. Add the rest of the ingredients, stir and simmer over medium heat for 35 minutes stirring from time to time.
3. Divide into bowls and serve for lunch.

Nutrition: calories 320, fat 12, carbs 12, protein 7

148. Bell Peppers Soup

Preparation time: 10 minutes

Cooking time: 40 minutes

Servings: 4

Ingredients:

- 4 shallots, chopped
- 3 carrots, chopped
- 1-pound mixed bell peppers, cut into strips
- A pinch of salt and black pepper
- 1 teaspoon hot paprika
- 4 cups water
- 1½ cups cauliflower florets, chopped
- 2 cups kale, chopped
- 2 tablespoons avocado oil
- 1 cup cherry tomatoes, chopped
- 1 teaspoon oregano, dried

Directions:

1. Heat up a pot with the oil over medium-high heat, add the shallots and carrots and cook for 5 minutes.
2. Add the peppers and the other ingredients, stir, simmer over medium heat for 35 minutes more, ladle into bowls and serve for lunch.

Nutrition: calories 210, fat 4.4, carbs 14, protein 6.3

149. Carrots and Onion Mix

Preparation time: 10 minutes

Cooking time: 25 minutes

Servings: 4

Ingredients:

- 1-pound baby carrots, trimmed
- 3 garlic cloves, minced

- 1 cup pearl onions, peeled
- Salt and black pepper to the taste
- 2 tablespoons coconut oil, melted
- 2 tablespoons chopped tarragon
- ¼ cup chopped parsley
- Juice of 1 lemon
- 1 tablespoon chopped thyme
- 1 cup cherry tomatoes, halved

Directions:

1. Heat up a pan with the oil over medium-high heat, add the onions and garlic and cook for 5 minutes.
2. Add the rest of the ingredients, stir, cook for 20 minutes more, divide between plates, and serve.

Nutrition: calories 173, fat 3, carbs 9, protein 5

150. Mixed Berry Crisp

Preparation Time: 10 Minutes

Cooking Time: 0

Servings: 4

Ingredients:

- 1 ½ cups mixed berries (I used raspberries, blueberries, and blackberries)
- ½ tablespoon cornstarch
- 2 tablespoons butter, room temperature
- ¼ cup old fashioned oats, plus 1 tablespoon old fashioned oats
- ¼ cup brown sugar
- 3 tablespoons flour
- ¼ teaspoon cinnamon
- ¼ teaspoon nutmeg
- 1 tablespoon water

Directions:

1. Preheat oven to 375 degrees.
2. In a small bowl, combine the butter, oats, brown sugar, flour, cinnamon, and nutmeg. Mix lightly with a fork until the mixture is crumbly.
3. Top the berries with the crisp mixture. Sprinkle the top of the crisp with water.
4. Bake for 25 minutes or until the fruit is bubbling and the topping is slightly browned.
5. Serve with ice cream, frozen yogurt, or whipped cream.

Nutrition: calories 226, fat 21, carbs 18, protein 11

151. Strawberry Daiquiri

Preparation Time: 10 Minutes

Cooking Time: 24 Minutes

Servings: 4

Ingredients:

- 1 (10-ounce) can frozen strawberry daiquiri concentrate
- 1 1/2 cups frozen strawberries
- 1 cup ice cube

Directions:

1. Combine all ingredients together in a blender until all the ice is crushed.
2. Add more or fewer ice cubes for the right texture.

Nutrition: calories 116, fat 21, carbs 8, protein 4

152. Virgin White Sangria

Preparation Time: 5 Minutes

Cooking Time: 4 Minutes

Servings: 1

Ingredients:

- 4 cups ocean spray white cranberry juice with Splenda

- 2 cups fresh fruit, sliced
- 1 cup diet lemon-lime soda
- 1 lime, juice of

Directions:

1. Combine all the ingredients except the soda in a large pitcher and chill for at least 1 hour.
2. When serving, add the soda. Serve with a pretty fruit garnish.

Nutrition: calories 129, fat 23, carbs 8, protein 18

153. Wow Cola Chicken

Preparation Time: 15 Minutes

Cooking Time: 14 Minutes

Servings: 1

Ingredients:

- 16 ounces boneless chicken breasts
- 1 (12 ounce) can diet cola
- 1 cup ketchup

Directions:

1. Place chicken in crockpot and then top with ketchup and then pour cola over all.
2. Cook on low for 6-8 hours.

Nutrition: calories 218, fat 19, carbs 18, protein 28

154. Warm Apple Delight

Preparation Time: 5 Minutes

Cooking Time: 4 Minutes

Servings: 1

Ingredients:

- 2 red apples, cored & cut in half
- 1 (375 ml) can flavored diet cola (cherry or strawberry suggested)

- 1 pinch Splenda sugar substitute or 1 pinch Equal sugar substitute
- 1 pinch cinnamon

Directions:

1. Place the apple in a baking dish, skin side down and pour the cola over.
2. Sprinkle with sweetener & cinnamon.
3. Bake in a pre-heated oven at 180.C for 25-30 minutes.

Nutrition: calories 156, fat 22, carbs 5, protein 4

155. Orange Dream Cake

Preparation Time: 5 Minutes

Cooking Time: 4 Minutes

Servings: 1

Ingredients:

- 2 egg whites
- 6 ounces sugar-free orange gelatin, divided (2 pkgs)
- 1 cup hot water
- 1 cup cold water

TOPPING

- 3 ½ ounces fat-free sugar-free vanilla pudding mix
- 1 cup nonfat milk
- 1 teaspoon vanilla extract
- 8 ounces Cool Whip Free, thawed

Directions

1. Mix Cake mix, soda, and egg whites together.
2. Pour batter into a 9 X 13-inch pan.
3. Bake as directed on box.
4. Pour gelatin mixture over top of the cake.
5. Refrigerate for 2 to 3 hours.

Nutrition: calories 109, fat 28, carbs 18, protein 19

156. Delicious Low-Cal Smoothie

Preparation Time: 5 Minutes

Cooking Time: 4 Minutes

Servings: 1

Ingredients:

- 1 cup frozen raspberries
- 1 1/2 cups frozen strawberries
- 1 cup pineapple
- 355 ml diet Sprite

Directions:

1. Blend on high power until smooth.
2. Serve in your favorite glasses, either with spoons or straws.

Nutrition: calories 126, fat 19, carbs 7, protein 11

Chapter 12

SNACKS & BREAD

157. Spinach and Sesame Crackers

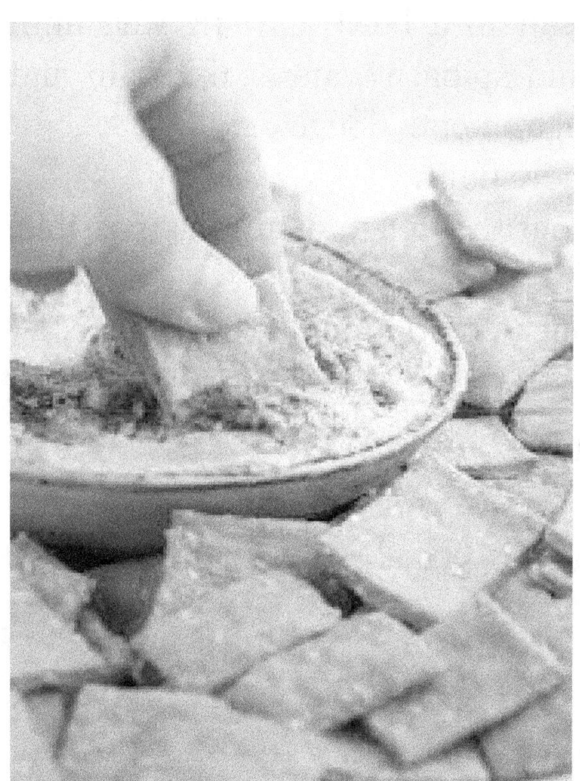

Preparation Time: 5 minutes

Cooking Time: 15 minutes

Servings: 4

Ingredients:

- 2 tablespoons white sesame seeds
- 1 cup fresh spinach, washed
- 1 2/3 cups of all-purpose flour
- 1/2 cup of water
- 1/2 teaspoon baking powder
- 1 teaspoon olive oil
- 1 teaspoon of salt

Directions:

1. Transfer the spinach to a blender with a half cup of water and blend until smooth.
2. Add 2 tablespoons white sesame seeds, ½ teaspoon baking powder, 1 2/3 cups all-purpose flour, and 1 teaspoon salt to a bowl and stir well until combined. Add in 1 teaspoon olive oil and spinach water. Mix again and knead by using your hands until you obtain a smooth dough.
3. If the made dough is too gluey, then add more flour.
4. Using your parchment paper lightly roll out the dough as thin as possible. Cut into squares with a pizza cutter.
5. Bake in a preheated oven at 400° for about 15to 20 minutes. Once done, let cool and then serve.

Nutrition: calories 190, fat 17, carbs 8, protein 11

158. Mini Nacho Pizzas

Preparation Time: 5 minutes

Cooking Time: 10 minutes

Servings: 4

Ingredients:

- 1/4 cup refried beans, vegan
- 2 tablespoons tomato, diced
- 2 English muffins, split in half
- 1/4 cup onion, sliced
- 1/3 cup vegan cheese, shredded

- 1 small jalapeno, sliced
- 1/3 cup roasted tomato salsa
- 1/2 avocado, diced and tossed in lemon juice

Directions:

1. Add the refried beans/salsa onto the muffin bread. Sprinkle with shredded vegan cheese followed by the veggie toppings.
2. Transfer to a baking sheet and place in a preheated oven at 350 to 400 F on a top rack.
3. Put into the oven for 10 minutes and then broil for 2minutes, so that the top becomes bubbly.
4. Take out from the oven and let them cool at room temperature.
5. Top with avocado. Enjoy!

Nutrition: calories 112, fat 23, carbs 18, protein 28

159. Pizza Sticks

Preparation Time: 10 minutes

Cooking Time: 30 minutes

Servings: 16 sticks

Ingredients:

- 5 tablespoons tomato sauce
- Few pinches of dried basil
- 1 block extra firm tofu
- 2 tablespoon + 2 teaspoon nutritional yeast

Directions:

1. Cape the tofu in a paper tissue and put a cutting board on top, place something heavy on top and drain for about 10 to 15 minutes.
2. In the meantime, line your baking sheet with parchment paper. Cut the tofu into 16 equal pieces and place them on a baking sheet.
3. Spread each pizza stick with a teaspoon of marinara sauce.
4. Sprinkle each stick with a half teaspoon of yeast, followed by basil on top.
5. Bake in a preheated oven at 425 F for about 28 to 30 minutes. Serve and enjoy!

Nutrition: calories 190, fat 23, carbs 8, protein 19

160. Raw Broccoli Poppers

Preparation Time: 2 minutes

Cooking Time: 8 minutes

Servings: 4

Ingredients:

- 1/8 cup of water
- 1/8 teaspoon of fine sea salt
- 4 cups broccoli florets, washed and cut into 1-inch pieces
- 1/4 teaspoon turmeric powder
- 1 cup unsalted cashews, soaked overnight or at least 3-4 hours and drained
- 1/4 teaspoon onion powder
- 1 red bell pepper, seeded and
- 2 heaping tablespoons nutritional
- 2 tablespoons lemon juice

Directions:

1. Transfer the drained cashews to a high-speed blender and pulse for about 30 seconds. Add in the chopped pepper and pulse again for 30 seconds.
2. Add some 2 tablespoons of lemon juice, 1/8 cup of water, 2 heaping tablespoons of nutritional yeast, ¼ teaspoon of onion powder, 1/8 teaspoon of fine sea salt, and 1/4 teaspoon of turmeric powder. Pulse for about 45 seconds until smooth.
3. Handover the broccoli into a bowl and add in chopped cheesy cashew mixture. Toss well until coated.
4. Transfer the pieces of broccoli to the trays of a yeast dehydrator.
5. Follow the dehydrator's instructions and dehydrate for about 8 minutes at 125 F or until crunchy.

Nutrition: calories 134, fat 18, carbs 6, protein 9

161. Blueberry Cauliflower

Preparation Time: 2 minutes

Cooking Time: 5 minutes

Servings: 1

Ingredients:

- ¼ cup of frozen strawberries
- 2 teaspoons maple syrup
- ¾ cup unsweetened cashew milk
- 1 teaspoon vanilla extract
- ½ cup of plain cashew yogurt
- 5 tablespoons powdered peanut butter
- ¾ cup of frozen wild blueberries
- ½ cup of cauliflower florets, coarsely chopped

Directions:

1. Add all the smoothie ingredients to a high-speed blender.
2. Blitz to combine until smooth.
3. Pour into a chilled glass and serve.

Nutrition: calories 219, fat 11, carbs 8, protein 17

162. Candied Ginger

Preparation Time: 10 minutes

Cooking Time: 40 minutes

Servings: 3 to 5

Ingredients:

- 2 1/2 cups salted pistachios, shelled
- 1 1/4 teaspoons powdered ginger
- 3 tablespoons pure maple syrup

Directions:

1. Add 1 1/4 teaspoons powdered ginger to a bowl with pistachios. Stir well until combined. There should be no lumps.

2. Drizzle with 3 tablespoons of maple syrup and stir well.
3. Transfer to a baking sheet lined with parchment paper and spread evenly.
4. Cook into a preheated oven at 275 F for about 20 minutes.
5. Take out from the oven, stir, and cook for a further 10 to 15 minutes.
6. Let it cool for about a few minutes until crispy. Enjoy!

163. Chia Crackers

Preparation Time: 20 minutes

Cooking Time: 1 hour

Servings: 24-26 crackers

Ingredients:

- 1/2 cup of pecans, chopped
- 1/2 cup of chia seeds
- 1/2 teaspoon cayenne pepper
- 1 cup of water
- 1/4 cup of nutritional yeast
- 1/2 cup of pumpkin seeds
- 1/4 cup of ground flax
- Salt and pepper, to taste

Directions:

1. Mix around 1/2 cup chia seeds and 1 cup water. Keep it aside.
2. Take another bowl and combine all the remaining ingredients. Combine well and stir in the chia water mixture until you obtain dough.
3. Transfer the dough onto a baking sheet and rollout (¼" thick).
4. Transfer into a preheated oven at 325ºF and bake for about half an hour.
5. Take out from the oven, flip over the dough, and cut it into the desired cracker shape/squares.
6. Spread and back again for a further half an hour, or until crispy and browned.
7. Once done, take out from the oven and let them cool at room temperature. Enjoy!

Nutrition: calories 90, fat 3, carbs 18, protein 10

164. Orange- Spiced Pumpkin Hummus

Preparation Time: 2 minutes

Cooking Time: 5 minutes

Servings: 4 cups

Ingredients:

- 1 tablespoon maple syrup
- 1/2 teaspoon salt
- 1 can (16oz.) garbanzo beans,
- 1/8 teaspoon ginger or nutmeg
- 1 cup of canned pumpkin
- 1/8 teaspoon cinnamon
- 1/4 cup of tahini
- 1 tablespoon fresh orange juice
- A pinch of orange zest, for garnish
- 1 tablespoon apple cider vinegar

Directions:

1. Mix all the ingredients to a food processor blender and blend until slightly chunky.
2. Serve right away and enjoy it!

165. Cinnamon Maple Sweet Potato Bites

Preparation Time: 5 minutes

Cooking Time: 25 minutes

Servings: 3 to 4

Ingredients:

- ½ teaspoon corn-starch
- 1 teaspoon cinnamon
- 4 medium sweet potatoes, then peeled, and cut into bite-size cubes
- 2 to 3 tablespoons maple syrup
- 3 tablespoons butter, melted

Directions:

1. Transfer the potato cubes to a Ziploc bag and add in 3 tablespoons of melted butter. Seal and shake well until the potato cubes are coated with butter.
2. Add in the remaining ingredients and shake again.
3. Transfer the potato cubes to a parchment-lined baking sheet. Cubes shouldn't be stacked on one another.
4. Sprinkle with cinnamon, if needed, and bake in a preheated oven at 425°F for about 25 to 30 minutes, stirring once during cooking.
5. Once done, take them out and stand at room temperature. Enjoy!

Nutrition: calories 188, fat 6, carbs 9, protein 18

166. Cheesy Kale Chips

Preparation Time: 3 minutes

Cooking Time: 12 minutes

Servings: 4

Ingredients:

- 3 tablespoons nutritional yeast
- 1 head curly kale, washed, ribs
- 3/4 teaspoon garlic powder
- 1 tablespoon olive oil
- 1 teaspoon onion powder
- Salt, to taste

Directions:

1. Line cookie sheets with parchment paper.
2. Drain the kale leaves and spread on a paper removed and leaves torn into a chip-towel. Then, kindly transfer the leaves to a bowl and sized pieces. Add in 1 teaspoon of onion powder, 3 tablespoons of nutritional yeast, 1 tablespoon of olive oil, and ¾ teaspoon of garlic powder. Mix with your hands.
3. Spread the kale onto prepared cookie sheets. They shouldn't touch each other.
4. Bake in a preheated oven for about 350 F for about 10 to 12 minutes.

5. Once crisp, take out from the oven, and sprinkle with a bit of salt. Serve and enjoy!

Nutrition: calories 286, fat 4, carbs 18, protein 10

167. Broccoli Bowls

Preparation time: 10 minutes

Cooking time: 15 minutes

Servings: 2

Ingredients:

- 1-pound broccoli florets
- 1 cup avocado, peeled, pitted, and cubed
- 1 red onion, chopped
- 1 red bell pepper, chopped
- 1 tablespoon coconut oil, melted
- 1 tablespoon avocado oil
- 1 teaspoon lemon juice
- Salt and black pepper to the taste
- ½ teaspoon ground turmeric

Directions:

1. Heat up a pan with the oil over medium heat, add the broccoli, avocado, and the other ingredients, stir and cook for 15 minutes.
2. Divide into bowls and serve as an appetizer.

Nutrition: calories 238, fat 8, carbs 10.3, protein 6.9

168. Celery Appetizer

Preparation time: 10 minutes

Cooking time: 30 minutes

Servings: 2

Ingredients:

- Juice of 1 lemon
- 6 celery stalks, chopped
- 2 teaspoons olive oil
- Salt and black pepper to the taste
- 4 tablespoons chopped parsley

Directions:

1. Spread the celery on a lined baking sheet, add the rest of the ingredients, toss, and cook at 390 degrees F for 30 minutes.
2. Serve as an appetizer.

Nutrition: calories 210, fat 6, carbs 6, protein 13

169. Seeds Mix

Preparation time: 10 minutes

Cooking time: 30 minutes

Servings: 4

Ingredients:

- 1 cup sunflower seeds
- 1 cup pumpkin seeds
- A pinch of salt and black pepper
- 1 teaspoon ground thyme
- A drizzle of olive oil

Directions:

1. Spread the seeds on a lined baking sheet, add the rest of the ingredients, toss, and bake at 350 degrees F for 30 minutes.
2. Serve as a snack.

Nutrition: calories 90, fat 2, carbs 1, protein 1

170. Herbed Endive Mix

Preparation time: 10 minutes

Cooking time: 10 minutes

Servings: 4

Ingredients:

- 2 tablespoons olive oil
- Salt and black pepper to the taste
- 2 tablespoons lime juice
- 3 endives, shredded
- 3 tablespoons chopped parsley
- 2 teaspoons chopped mint
- 1 tablespoon chopped tarragon

Directions:

1. On a lined baking sheet, mix the endives with the rest of the ingredients and toss.
2. Bake in the oven at 400 degrees F for 10 minutes.
3. Serve as an appetizer.

Nutrition: calories 160, fat 7, carbs 3, protein 3

171. Beet Chips

Preparation time: 10 minutes

Cooking time: 45 minutes

Servings: 4

Ingredients:

- 2 big beets, peeled and thinly sliced
- Juice of 1 lemon
- 1 Serrano chili pepper, chopped
- ½ teaspoon fresh grated ginger
- ¼ teaspoon minced garlic
- A pinch of salt and black pepper

- 2 tablespoons avocado oil
- ¼ cup chopped cilantro

Directions:

1. Spread the chips on a lined baking sheet, add the rest of the ingredients, toss, and bake at 390 degrees F for 45 minutes.
2. Serve as a snack.

Nutrition: calories 160, fat 3, carbs 5, protein 5

172. Avocado and Radish Salsa

Preparation time: 10 minutes

Cooking time: 0 minutes

Servings: 4

Ingredients:

- 2 small avocados, pitted, peeled, and chopped
- 2 cups radishes, cubed
- 1 cup cucumber, cubed
- Juice of 1 lemon
- 1 tablespoon avocado oil
- 1 tablespoon chives, chopped
- 1 tablespoon cilantro, chopped

Directions:

1. In a bowl, mix the avocados with the radishes and the other ingredients, toss, and serve.

Nutrition: calories 220, fat 6, carbs 12, protein 6

173. Tomato Platter

Preparation time: 10 minutes

Cooking time: 20 minutes

Servings: 6

Ingredients:

- 2 pounds cherry tomatoes, halved
- 1 teaspoon crushed red pepper flakes
- 3 garlic cloves, minced
- 1 handful chopped parsley
- 1 teaspoon curry powder
- 1 teaspoon sweet paprika
- Salt and black pepper to the taste
- 1 tablespoon avocado oil

Directions:

1. Spread the tomatoes on a lined baking sheet, add the rest of the ingredients, toss and roast at 400 degrees F for 20 minutes.
2. Serve as an appetizer.

Nutrition: calories 170, fat 3.4, carbs 6, protein 5.5

174. Cauliflower and Broccoli Bites

Preparation time: 10 minutes

Cooking time: 20 minutes

Servings: 4

Ingredients:

- 1 cup cauliflower florets
- 1 cup broccoli florets
- 2 tablespoons avocado oil
- 2 tablespoons green onions, chopped
- 1 teaspoon sweet paprika
- 1 tablespoon lemon juice
- A pinch of salt

Directions:

1. Spread the broccoli and cauliflower on a lined baking sheet, add the rest of the ingredients, toss, and bake at 400 degrees F for 20 minutes.
2. Divide into bowls and serve as a snack.

Nutrition: calories 180, fat 6.6, carbs 6, protein 5.2

175. Avocado Bites

Preparation time: 10 minutes

Cooking time: 0 minutes

Servings: 2

Ingredients:

- 2 avocados, peeled, pitted, and cubed
- 2 tablespoons sweet paprika
- juice of 1 lemon
- 1 teaspoon basil, dried
- 1 teaspoon oregano, dried
- Salt and black pepper to the taste
- 1 tablespoon olive oil

Directions:

1. In a bowl, mix the avocado bites with the paprika and the other ingredients, toss, divide into bowls and serve as a snack.

Nutrition: calories 60, fat 3, carbs 4.2, protein 4.4

176. Chives Dip

Preparation time: 10 minutes

Cooking time: 0 minutes

Servings: 4

Ingredients:

- 2 cups chives, chopped
- 1/2 cup almond milk
- ¼ cup chopped carrot
- ¼ cup chopped red onion
- Salt and black pepper to the taste
- 1 teaspoon sweet paprika

Directions:

1. In a blender, mix the chives with the carrot and the other ingredients and blend well.
2. Divide into bowls and serve.

Nutrition: calories 210, fat 3.4, carbs 6.4, protein 6

177. Stuffed Avocado

Preparation time: 10 minutes

Cooking time: 0 minutes

Servings: 2

Ingredients:

- 2 avocados, halved, pitted and flesh scooped out
- ¼ cup chives, chopped
- ½ cup carrot, grated
- ½ cup kale, chopped
- 1 teaspoon dried thyme
- A pinch of salt and black pepper
- ¼ teaspoon cayenne pepper
- 1 teaspoon paprika
- Salt and black pepper to the taste
- 2 tablespoons lemon juice

Directions:

1. In a bowl, mix the chives with carrots, avocado flesh, and the other ingredients except for the avocado shells and stir well.
2. Stuff the avocado skins with this mix, arrange them on a platter, and serve as an appetizer.

Nutrition: calories 160, fat 10, carbs 4,2, protein 5.5

178. Radish Chips

Preparation time: 10 minutes

Cooking time: 20 minutes

Servings: 4

Ingredients:

- 2 teaspoons avocado oil
- 15 radishes, sliced
- A pinch of salt and black pepper
- 1 tablespoon chopped chives

Directions:

1. Arrange radish slices on a lined baking sheet, add the other ingredients, toss, and place in the oven at 375 degrees F.
2. Bake for 10 minutes on each side, divide into bowls, and serve cold.

Nutrition: calories 30, fat 1, fiber 2, carbs 7, protein 1

179. Avocado Cream

Preparation time: 10 minutes

Cooking time: 10 minutes

Servings: 4

Ingredients:

- 2 avocados, pitted, peeled, and chopped
- 1 cup almond milk
- 2 scallions, chopped
- Salt and black pepper to the taste
- 2 tablespoons coconut oil
- 1 tablespoon chives, chopped

Directions:

1. Heat up a pot with the coconut oil over medium heat.
2. Add scallions and avocado and cook for 2 minutes.

3. Add the rest of the ingredients, cook for 8 minutes more, blend with an immersion blender, divide into bowls, and serve.

Nutrition: calories 162, fat 4.4, carbs 6, protein 6

180. Chives Chutney

Preparation time: 10 minutes

Cooking time: 20 minutes

Servings: 10

Ingredients:

- 1 teaspoon cumin seeds
- 1 tablespoon avocado oil
- 1 cup chives, chopped
- ½ cup water
- 1 cup cherry tomatoes, cubed
- ½ teaspoon garam masala
- 1 teaspoon ground ginger
- ½ teaspoon cayenne pepper

Directions:

1. Heat up a pan with the oil over medium heat, add the chives and cumin and cook for 5 minutes.
2. Add the rest of the ingredients, simmer the mixture over medium heat for 15 minutes more, divide into bowls, and serve cold.

Nutrition: calories 120, fat 4,4, carbs 5, protein 6

181. Onion Bowls

Preparation time: 10 minutes

Cooking time: 15 minutes

Servings: 4

Ingredients:

- 1 tablespoon avocado oil
- 3 red onions, cut into thin strips
- A pinch of salt and black pepper
- 1 teaspoon sweet paprika
- 1 teaspoon dried basil
- 1 teaspoon oregano, dried

Directions:

1. Heat up a pan with the oil over medium heat, add the onions and cook for 5 minutes.
2. Add the rest of the ingredients, stir, cook for 10 minutes more, divide into bowls, and serve as a snack

Nutrition: calories 127, fat 4, carbs 6, protein 4.4

182. Chia Crackers

Preparation time: 10 minutes

Cooking time: 35 minutes

Servings: 12

Ingredients:

- 1 cup ice water
- 1 cup ground chia seeds
- 2 tablespoons avocado oil
- 2 tablespoons flaxseeds
- ¼ teaspoon dried oregano
- ¼ teaspoon turmeric powder
- ¼ teaspoon sweet paprika
- Salt and black pepper to the taste
- ¼ teaspoon basil, dried

Directions:

1. In a bowl, mix chia seeds with the rest of the ingredients.
2. Stir until you obtain a firm mix then spread it on a baking sheet and place in the oven at 350 degrees F and bake for 35 minutes.
3. Remove from the oven and set aside to cool down.
4. Cut into medium crackers and serve as a snack.

Nutrition: calories 50, fat 3, carbs 5, protein 2

183. Cilantro Guacamole

Preparation time: 3 hours

Cooking time: 0 minutes

Servings: 4

Ingredients:

- 2 avocados, pitted, peeled, and chopped
- ½ cup chopped cilantro
- Juice and zest of 1 lemon
- 1 cup almond milk

Directions:

1. In a blender, mix the avocados with cilantro and the other ingredients, blend and serve.

Nutrition: calories 150, fat 7, carbs 8, protein 4

Chapter 13

LUNCH AND ENTRÉES

184. Green Bean Casserole

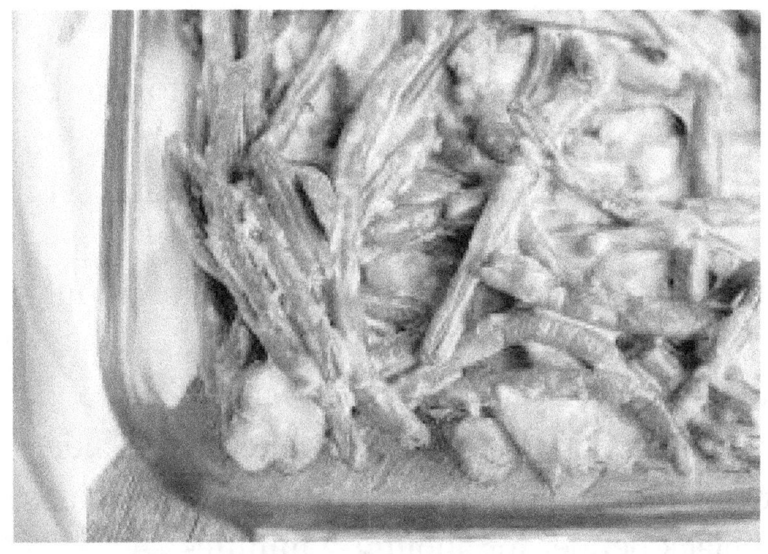

Preparation time: 20 minutes

Cooking Time: 20 minutes.

Servings: 6

Ingredients:

For Onion Slices:

- ½ cup yellow onion, sliced very thinly
- ¼ cup almond flour
- 1/8 tsp garlic powder

- Sea salt and freshly ground black pepper, to taste

For Casserole:

- 1 lb. fresh green beans, trimmed
- 1 tbsp olive oil
- 8 oz fresh cremini mushrooms, sliced
- ½ cup yellow onion, sliced thinly
- 1/8 tsp garlic powder
- Sea salt and freshly ground black pepper, to taste
- 1 tsp fresh thyme, chopped
- ½ cup homemade vegetable broth
- ½ cup coconut cream

Directions:

2. Preheat the oven to 350 degrees F.
3. For onion slices, place all the ingredients in a bowl and toss them to coat the onion well.
4. Arrange the onion slices onto a large baking sheet in a single layer and set it aside.
5. In a pan of salted boiling water, add the green beans and cook for about 5 minutes.
6. Drain the green beans and transfer them into a bowl of ice water.
7. Again, drain well and transfer them again into a large bowl. Set them aside.
8. In a large skillet, heat oil over medium-high heat and sauté the mushrooms, onion, garlic powder, salt, and black pepper for about 2-3 minutes.
9. Stir in the thyme and broth and cook for about 3-5 minutes or until all the liquid is absorbed.
10. Remove from the heat and transfer the mushroom mixture into the bowl with the green beans.
11. Add the coconut cream and stir to combine well.
12. Transfer the mixture into a 10-inch casserole dish.
13. Place the casserole dish and baking sheet of onion slices into the oven.
14. Bake for about 15-17 minutes.
15. Remove the baking dish and sheet from the oven and let it cool for about 5 minutes before serving.

16. Top the casserole with the crispy onion slices evenly.
17. Cut into 6 equal-sized portions and serve.

Nutrition: calories 190, fat 2, carbs 18, protein 32

185. Vegetarian Pie

Preparation time: 20 minutes

Cooking Time: 1 hour 20 minutes

Servings: 8

Ingredients:

For Topping:

- 5 cups water
- 1¼ cups yellow cornmeal

For Filing:

- 1 tbsp extra-virgin olive oil
- 1 large onion, chopped
- 1 medium red bell pepper, seeded and chopped
- 2 garlic cloves, minced
- 1 tsp dried oregano, crushed
- 2 tsp chili powder
- 2 cups fresh tomatoes, chopped
- 2½ cups cooked pinto beans
- 2 cups boiled corn kernels

Directions:

1. Preheat the oven to 375 degrees F. Lightly grease a shallow baking dish.
2. In a pan, add the water over medium-high heat and bring to a boil.
3. Slowly, add the cornmeal, stirring continuously.
4. Reduce the heat to low and cook covered for about 20 minutes, stirring occasionally.
5. Meanwhile, prepare the filling. In a large skillet, heat the oil over medium heat and sauté the onion and bell pepper for about 3-4 minutes.
6. Add the garlic, oregano, and spices and sauté for about 1 minute

7. Add the remaining ingredients and stir to combine.
8. Reduce the heat to low and simmer for about 10-15 minutes, stirring occasionally.
9. Remove from the heat.
10. Place half of the cooked cornmeal into the prepared baking dish evenly.
11. Place the filling mixture over the cornmeal evenly.
12. Place the remaining cornmeal over the filling mixture evenly.
13. Bake for 45-50 minutes or until the top becomes golden brown.
14. Remove the pie from the oven and set it aside for about 5 minutes before serving.

Nutrition: calories 176, fat 1, carbs 10, protein 22

186. Rice & Lentil Loaf

Preparation time: 20 minutes

Cooking Time: 1 hour 50 minutes

Servings: 8

Ingredients:

- 1¾ cups plus 2 tbsp filtered water, divided
- ½ cup wild rice
- ½ cup brown lentils
- Pinch of sea salt
- ½ tsp no-sodium Italian seasoning
- 1 medium yellow onion, chopped
- 1 celery stalk, chopped
- 6 cremini mushrooms, chopped
- 4 garlic cloves, minced
- ¾ cup rolled oats
- ½ cup pecans, chopped finely
- ¾ cup homemade tomato sauce
- ½ tsp red pepper flakes, crushed
- 1 tsp fresh rosemary, minced
- 2 tsp fresh thyme, minced

Directions:

1. In a pan, add 1¾ cups of water, rice, lentils, salt, and Italian seasoning and bring them to a boil over medium-high heat.
2. Reduce the heat to low and simmer covered for about 45 minutes.
3. Remove from the heat and set it aside still covered for at least 10 minutes.
4. Preheat the oven to 350 degrees F.
5. With parchment paper, line a 9x5-inch loaf pan.
6. In a skillet, heat the remaining water over medium heat and sauté the onion, celery, mushrooms, and garlic for about 4-5 minutes.
7. Remove from the heat and let it cool slightly.
8. In a large mixing bowl, add the oats, pecans, tomato sauce, and fresh herbs and mix until well combined.
9. Combine the rice mixture and vegetable mixture with the oat mixture and mix well.
10. In a blender, add the mixture and pulse until a chunky mixture forms.
11. Transfer the mixture into the prepared loaf pan evenly.
12. With a piece of foil, cover the loaf pan and bake it for about 40 minutes.
13. Uncover and bake for about 15-20 minutes more or until the top becomes golden brown.
14. Remove it from the oven and set it aside for about 5-10 minutes before slicing.
15. Cut into desired sized slices and serve.

Nutrition: calories 220, fat 3, carbs 8, protein 21

187. Quinoa & Chickpea Salad

Preparation time: 15 minutes

Cooking time: 45 minutes

Servings: 8

Ingredients:

- 1¾ cups homemade vegetable broth
- 1 cup quinoa, rinsed
- Sea salt, to taste
- 1½ cups cooked chickpeas

- 1 medium green bell pepper, seeded and chopped
- 1 medium red bell pepper, seeded and chopped
- 2 cucumbers, chopped
- ½ cup scallion (green part only), chopped
- 1 tablespoon olive oil
- 2 tablespoons fresh cilantro leaves, chopped

Directions:

1. In a pan, add the broth and bring to a boil over high heat.
2. Add the quinoa and salt and cook until boiling again.
3. Reduce the heat to low and simmer covered for about 15-20 minutes or until all the liquid is absorbed.
4. Remove from the heat and set aside still covered for about 5-10 minutes.
5. Uncover and fluff the quinoa with a fork.
6. In a large serving bowl, add the quinoa and the remaining ingredients and gently toss to coat.
7. Serve immediately.

Nutrition: calories 276, fat 3, carbs 18, protein 28

188. Mixed Veggie Soup

Preparation time: 20 minutes

Cooking Time: 20 minutes.

Servings: 6

Ingredients:

- 1½ tablespoons olive oil
- 4 medium carrots, peeled and chopped
- 1 medium onion, chopped
- 2 garlic cloves, minced
- 2 celery stalks, chopped
- 2 cups fresh tomatoes, chopped finely
- 3 cups small cauliflower florets
- 3 cups small broccoli florets
- 3 cups frozen peas

- 8 cups homemade vegetable broth
- 3 tablespoons fresh lemon juice
- Sea salt, to taste

Directions:

1. In a large soup pan, heat the oil over medium heat and sauté the carrots, celery, and onion for 6 minutes.
2. Stir in the garlic and sauté for about 1 minute.
3. Add the tomatoes and cook for about 2-3 minutes, crushing them with the back of a spoon.
4. Add the vegetables and broth and bring to a boil over high heat.
5. Reduce the heat to low.
6. Cover the pan and simmer for about 30-35 minutes.
7. Mix in the lemon juice and salt and remove from the heat.
8. Serve hot.

Nutrition: calories 173, fat 5, carbs 18, protein 19

189. Beans & Barley Soup

Preparation time: 15 minutes

Cooking time: 40 minutes

Servings: 4

Ingredients:

- 1 tablespoon olive oil
- 1 white onion, chopped
- 2 celery stalks, chopped
- 1 large carrot, peeled and chopped
- 2 tablespoons fresh rosemary, chopped
- 2 garlic cloves, minced
- 4 cups fresh tomatoes, chopped
- 4 cups homemade vegetable broth
- 1 cup pearl barley
- 2 cups cooked white beans
- 2 tablespoons fresh lemon juice

- 4 tablespoons fresh parsley leaves, chopped

Directions:

1. In a large soup pan, heat the oil over medium heat and sauté the onion, celery, and carrot for about 4-5 minutes.
2. Add the garlic and rosemary and sauté for about 1 minute.
3. Add the tomatoes and cook for 3-4 minutes, crushing them with the back of a spoon.
4. Add the barley and broth and bring to a boil.
5. Reduce the heat to low and simmer covered for about 20-25 minutes.
6. Stir in the beans and lemon juice and simmer for about 5 minutes more.
7. Garnish with parsley and serve hot

Nutrition: calories 278, fat 13, carbs 8, protein 19

190. Tofu & Bell Pepper Stew

Preparation time: 15 minutes

Cooking time: 15 minutes

Servings: 6

Ingredients:

- 2 tablespoons garlic
- 1 jalapeño pepper, seeded and chopped
- 1 (16-ounce) jar roasted red peppers, rinsed, drained, and chopped
- 2 cups homemade vegetable broth
- 2 cups filtered water
- 1 medium green bell pepper, seeded and sliced thinly
- 1 medium red bell pepper, seeded and sliced thinly
- 1 (16-ounce) package extra-firm tofu, drained and cubed
- 1 (10-ounce) package frozen baby spinach, thawed

Directions:

1. Add the garlic, jalapeño pepper, and roasted red peppers in a food processor and pulse until smooth.

2. In a large pan, add the puree, broth, and water and cook until boiling over medium-high heat.
3. Add the bell peppers and tofu and stir to combine.
4. Reduce the heat to medium and cook for about 5 minutes.
5. Stir in the spinach and cook for about 5 minutes.
6. Serve hot.

Nutrition: calories 111, fat 7, carbs 9, protein 18

191. Lentils with Kale

Preparation time: 15 minutes

Cooking time: 20 minutes

Servings: 6

Ingredients:

- 1½ cups red lentils
- 1½ cups homemade vegetable broth
- 1½ tablespoons olive oil
- ½ cup onion, chopped
- 1 teaspoon fresh ginger, peeled and minced
- 2 garlic cloves, minced
- 1½ cups tomato, chopped
- 6 cups fresh kale, tough ends removed and chopped
- Sea salt and ground black pepper, to taste

Directions:

1. In a pan, add the broth and lentils and bring to a boil over medium-high heat.
2. Reduce the heat to low and simmer covered for about 20 minutes or until almost all the liquid is absorbed.
3. Remove from the heat and set aside still covered.
4. Meanwhile, in a large skillet, heat oil over medium heat and sauté the onion for about 5-6 minutes.
5. Add the ginger and garlic and sauté for about 1 minute.
6. Add tomatoes and kale and cook for about 4-5 minutes.

7. Stir in the lentils, salt, and black pepper then remove from heat.
8. Serve hot.

Nutrition: calories 188, fat 4, carbs 6, protein 11

192. Veggie Ratatouille

Preparation time: 20 minutes

Cooking time: 45 minutes 5 minutes

Servings: 4

Ingredients:

- 6 ounces homemade tomato paste
- 3 tablespoons olive oil, divided
- ½ of an onion, chopped
- 3 tablespoons garlic, minced
- Sea salt and freshly ground black pepper, to taste
- ¾ cup filtered water
- 1 eggplant, sliced into thin circles
- 1 red bell pepper, seeded and sliced into thin circles
- 1 yellow bell pepper, seeded and sliced into thin circles
- 1 tablespoon fresh thyme leaves, minced
- 1 tablespoon fresh lemon juice

Directions:

1. Preheat oven to 375 degrees F.
2. In a bowl, add the tomato paste, 1 tablespoon of oil, onion, garlic, salt, and black pepper and mix nicely.
3. In the bottom of a 10x10-inch baking dish, spread the tomato paste mixture evenly.
4. Arrange alternating vegetable slices starting at the outer edge of the baking dish and working concentrically towards the center.
5. Drizzle the remaining oil and lemon juice over the vegetables and sprinkle them with salt and black pepper followed by the thyme.
6. Arrange a piece of parchment paper over the vegetables.
7. Bake for about 45 minutes.

8. Serve hot.

Nutrition: calories 143, fat 4, carbs 7, protein 19

193. Baked Beans

Preparation time: 15 minutes

Cooking time: 2 hours 5 minutes

Servings: 4

Ingredients:

- ¼ pound dry lima beans, soaked overnight and drained
- ¼ pound dry red kidney beans, soaked overnight and drained
- 1¼ tablespoons olive oil
- 1 small yellow onion, chopped
- 4 garlic cloves, minced
- 1 teaspoon dried thyme, crushed
- ½ teaspoon ground cumin
- ½ teaspoon red pepper flakes, crushed
- ¼ teaspoon smoked paprika
- 1 tablespoon fresh lemon juice
- 1 cup homemade tomato sauce
- 1 cup homemade vegetable broth

Directions:

1. Add the beans to a large pan of boiling water and bring back to a boil.
2. Reduce the heat to low.
3. Cover the pan and cook for about 1 hour.
4. Drain the beans well.
5. Preheat the oven to 325 degrees F.
6. In a large oven-proof pan, heat the oil over medium heat and sauté the onion for about 4 minutes.
7. Add the garlic, thyme, and spices, and sauté for about 1 minute.
8. Stir in the cooked beans and remaining ingredients and immediately remove from the heat.
9. Cover the pan and bake in oven for about 1 hour.

10. Serve hot.

Nutrition: calories 160, fat 2, carbs 7, protein 19

194. Cannellini Bean Cashew Dip

Preparation time: 1 hour

Cooking time: 1 hour

Servings: 8

Ingredients:

- 1 15-ounce can cannellini beans, rinsed and drained
- ½ cup raw cashews
- 1 clove garlic, smashed
- 2 tablespoons diced, red bell pepper
- ½ teaspoon sea salt
- ¼ teaspoon cayenne pepper
- 4 teaspoons lemon juice
- 2 tablespoons water
- Dill sprigs or weed for garnish

Directions:

1. Place the beans, cashews, garlic, and bell pepper in the food processor and pulse several times to break it up.
2. Add the salt, cayenne, lemon juice, and water and process until smooth.
3. Scrape into a bowl, cover, and refrigerate for at least an hour before serving.
4. Garnish with fresh dill and serve with vegetables, crackers, or pita chips.

Nutrition: calories 132, fat 6, carbs 9, protein 18

195. Cauliflower Popcorn

Preparation time: 1 day and 1 hour

Cooking time: 1 day

Servings: 2

Ingredients:

- ¼ cup sun-dried tomatoes
- ¾ cup dates
- 2 heads cauliflower
- ½ cup water
- 2 tablespoons raw tahini
- 1 tablespoon apple cider vinegar
- 2 teaspoons onion powder
- 2 teaspoons garlic powder
- 1 teaspoon ground cayenne pepper
- 2 tablespoons nutritional yeast (optional)

Directions:

1. Cover the sun-dried tomatoes with warm water and let them soak for an hour.
2. If the dates are not soft and fresh, soak them in warm water for an hour in another bowl.
3. Cut the cauliflower into very small, bite-sized pieces then set aside.
4. Put the drained tomatoes and dates in a blender along with the water, tahini, apple cider vinegar, onion powder, garlic powder, cayenne pepper, nutritional yeast, and turmeric. Blend into a thick, smooth consistency.
5. Pour this mixture into the bowl, atop the cauliflower, and mix so that all the pieces are coated.
6. Place the cauliflower in the dehydrator and spread it out to make a single layer. Sprinkle with a little sea salt and set for 115 degrees, Fahrenheit for 12 to 24 hours or until it becomes exactly as crunchy as you like it. I let mine go for 15 to 16 hours, but the time will vary based on your taste preference as well as the ambient humidity.
7. Store in an airtight container until serving.

Nutrition: calories 170, fat 2, carbs 6, protein 16

196. Cinnamon Apple Chips with Dip

Preparation time: 3 hours and 30 minutes

Cooking time: 3 hours

Servings: 2

Ingredients:

- 1 cup raw cashews
- 2 apples, thinly sliced
- 1 lemon
- 1½ cups water, divided
- Cinnamon plus more to dust the chips
- Another medium cored apple quartered
- 1 tablespoon honey or agave
- 1 teaspoon cinnamon
- ¼ teaspoon sea salt

Directions:

1. Place the cashews in a bowl of warm water, deep enough to cover them, and let them soak overnight.
2. Preheat the oven to 200 degrees, Fahrenheit. Line two baking sheets with parchment paper.
3. Juice the lemon into a large glass bowl and add two cups of the water. Place the sliced apples in the water as you cut them and when done, swish them around and drain.
4. Spread the apple slices across the baking sheet in a single layer and sprinkle with a little cinnamon. Bake for 90 minutes.
5. Remove the slices from the oven and flip each of them over. Put them back in the oven and bake for another 90 minutes, or until they are crisp. Remember, they will get crisper as they cool.
6. While the apple slices are cooking, drain the cashews and put them in a blender, along with the quartered apple, the honey, a teaspoon of cinnamon, and a half cup of the remaining water. Process until thick and creamy. I like

to refrigerate my dip for about an hour to chill before serving alongside the room temperature apple slices.

Nutrition: calories 190, fat 1, carbs 18, protein 32

197. Crunchy Asparagus Spears

Preparation time: 25 minutes

Cooking time: 25 minutes

Servings: 4

Ingredients:

- 1 bunch asparagus spears (about 12 spears)
- ¼ cup nutritional yeast
- 2 tablespoons hemp seeds
- 1 teaspoon garlic powder
- ¼ teaspoon paprika (or more if you like paprika)
- ⅛ teaspoon ground pepper
- ¼ cup whole-wheat breadcrumbs
- Juice of ½ lemon

Directions:

1. Preheat the oven to 350 degrees, Fahrenheit. Line a baking sheet with parchment paper.
2. Wash the asparagus, snapping off the white part at the bottom. Save it for making vegetable stock.
3. Mix together the nutritional yeast, hemp seed, garlic powder, paprika, pepper, and breadcrumbs.
4. Place asparagus spears on the baking sheets giving them a little room in between and sprinkle with the mixture in the bowl.
5. Bake for up to 25 minutes, until crispy.
6. Serve with lemon juice if desired.

Nutrition: calories 156, fat 4, carbs 7, protein 18

198. Cucumber Bites with Chive and Sunflower Seeds

Preparation time: 5 minutes

Cooking time: 5 minutes

Servings: 2

Ingredients:

- 1 cup raw sunflower seed
- ½ teaspoon salt
- ½ cup chopped fresh chives
- 1 clove garlic, chopped
- 2 tablespoons red onion, minced
- 2 tablespoons lemon juice
- ½ cup water (might need more or less)
- 4 large cucumbers

Directions:

1. Place the sunflower seeds and salt in the food processor and process to a fine powder. It will take only about 10 seconds.
2. Add the chives, garlic, onion, lemon juice, and water and process until creamy, scraping down the sides frequently. The mixture should be very creamy; if not, add a little more water.
3. Cut the cucumbers into 1½-inch coin-like pieces.
4. Spread a spoonful of the sunflower mixture on top and set on a platter. Sprinkle more chopped chives on top and refrigerate until ready to serve.

Nutrition: calories 177, fat 1, carbs 8, protein 16

199. Garlicky Kale Chips

Preparation time: 1 hour and 30 min

Cooking time: 1 hour

Servings: 2

Ingredients:

- 4 cloves garlic
- 1 cup olive oil
- 8 to 10 cups fresh kale, chopped
- 1 tablespoon of garlic-flavored olive oil
- ½ teaspoon garlic salt
- ½ teaspoon pepper
- 1 pinch red pepper flakes (optional)

Directions:

1. Peel and crush the garlic clove and place it in a small jar with a lid. Pour the olive oil over the top, cover tightly, and shake. This will keep in the refrigerator for several days. When you're ready to use it, strain out the garlic and retain the oil.
2. Preheat the oven to 175 degrees, Fahrenheit.
3. Spread out the kale on a baking sheet and drizzle with the olive oil. Sprinkle with garlic salt, pepper, and red pepper flakes.
4. Bake for an hour, remove from the oven, and let the chips cool.
5. Store in an airtight container if you don't plan to eat them right away.

Nutrition: calories 211, fat 3, carbs 18, protein 21

200. Hummus-Stuffed Baby Potatoes

Preparation time: 30 minutes

Cooking time: 30 minutes

Servings: 2

Ingredients:

- 12 small red potatoes, walnut-sized or slightly larger
- Hummus
- 2 green onions, thinly sliced
- ¼ teaspoon paprika, for garnish

Directions:

1. Place two to three inches of water in a saucepan, set a steamer inside, and bring the water to a boil.
2. Place the whole potatoes in the steamer basket and steam for about 20 minutes or until soft. Keep the pan from boiling dry by adding additional hot water as needed.
3. Dump the potatoes into a colander and run cold water over them until they can be handled.
4. Cut each potato open and scoop out most of the pulp, leaving the skin and a thin layer of potato intact.
5. Mix the hummus with most of the green onions (keep enough for garnish) and spoon a little into the area where the potato has been scooped out.
6. Sprinkle each filled potato half with paprika and serve.

Nutrition: calories 329, fat 3, carbs 8, protein 14

HOW MUCH YOU MUST DRINK AND WHY IT IS SO IMPORTANT

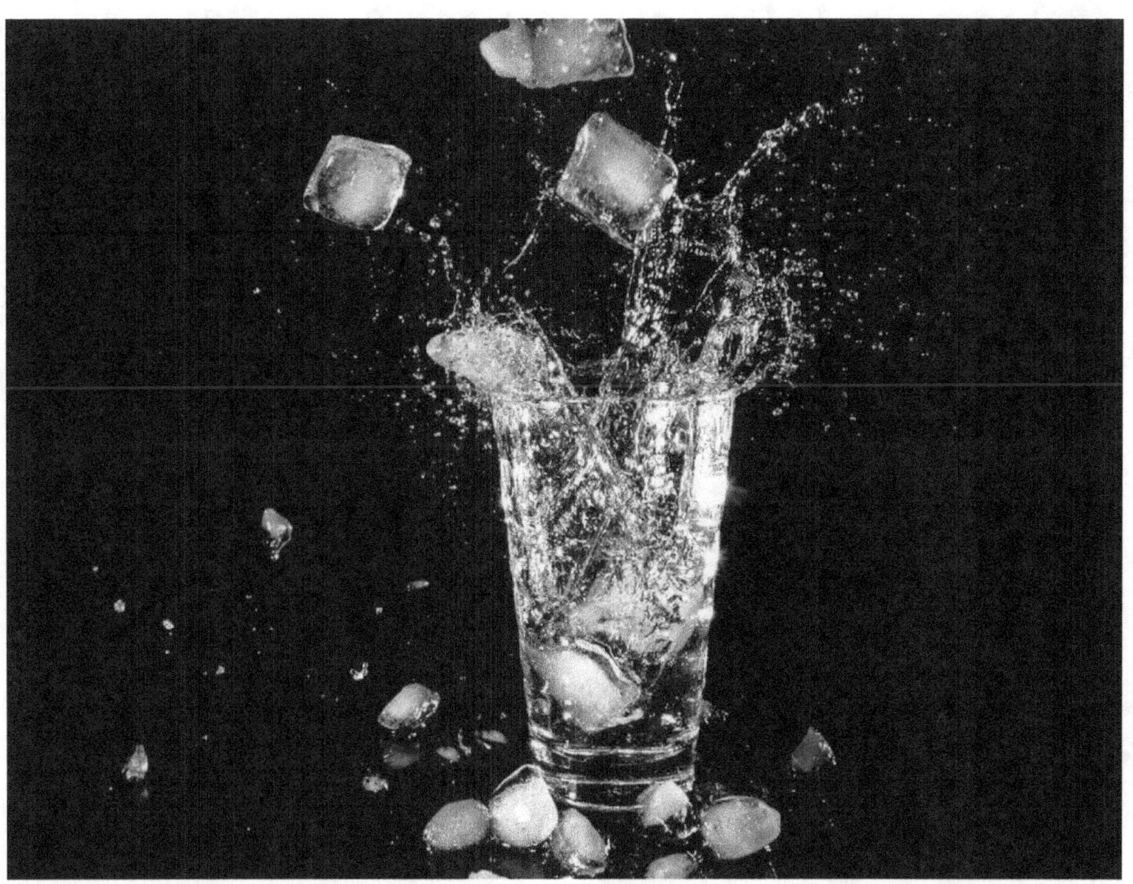

Enough liquid in the body, especially warm liquid, can help drain the sinuses and thin the mucus. Thus, drinking large amounts of water can help clear out mucus from the body. Dr. Sebi recommends a high intake of water. Also, most fruits and vegetables recommended by Dr. Sebi's diet have high water content. These foods help to keep the body hydrated and prevent excess mucus production.

Moreover, some drinks like coffee and alcohol can cause dehydration in the body. Anyone on the Dr. Sebi diet must stay away from alcohol. This helps to avoid dehydration.

Action: Take a lot of water, smoothies, and juice made with Dr. Sebi's approved foods.

Expectorants

Expectorants are known to help in clearing mucus. Expectorants loosen and thin mucus, which makes it easy to cough it out of the system. There are some herbs in the Dr. Sebi diet which can serve as expectorants. The most used herb of Dr. Sebi's approved herbs is the Red Clover.

Red Clover is a super healthy herb which aids circulation in the body. It is a natural blood purifier, and also serves as an expectorant. It is widely used by women in treating menopause-related conditions like hot flashes and lumbar spine protection. So, taking red clover can help to loosen and clear mucus from the body.

Action: In 8 oz of hot water, steep 1 - 2 teaspoons of the dried flower and allow for up to 30 minutes. Then drink at least 2 and not more than 3 cups per day. Or, sip 1ml of the fluid extract with hot water three times daily.

Essential Oils

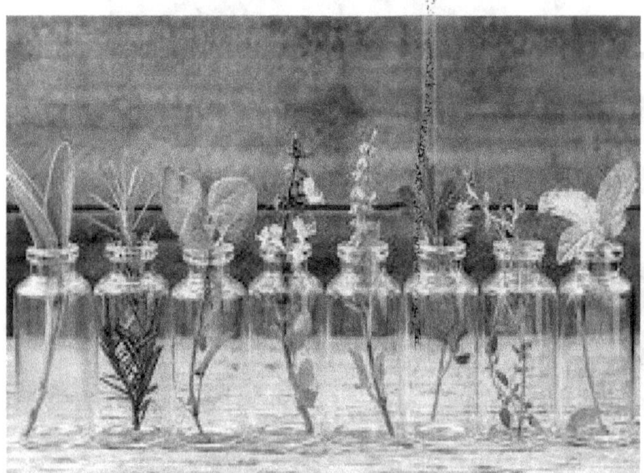

Some essential oils have been proposed to be very effective in the treatment of lung disease-related symptoms. People use essential oils for the treatment and prevention of chest cold and sinusitis. Some of these essential oils can be gotten from Dr. Sebi approved products like eucalyptus, oregano, and thyme.

Eucalyptus has been widely used for many years to treat coughs and reduce mucus production. It helps to loosen the mucus so it can be easily coughed out. Thus, it relieves nagging coughs.

Action: Make your own homemade vapor rub by adding 12 drops of eucalyptus oil to ¼ cup of coconut oil. Alternatively, add 1 drop of eucalyptus oil to 1 teaspoon of water.

First test the mixture to know whether it is safe for use. Then apply it directly on your skin, especially on your throat and chest. This makes the scents easily reach the nose and mouth.

CONCLUSION

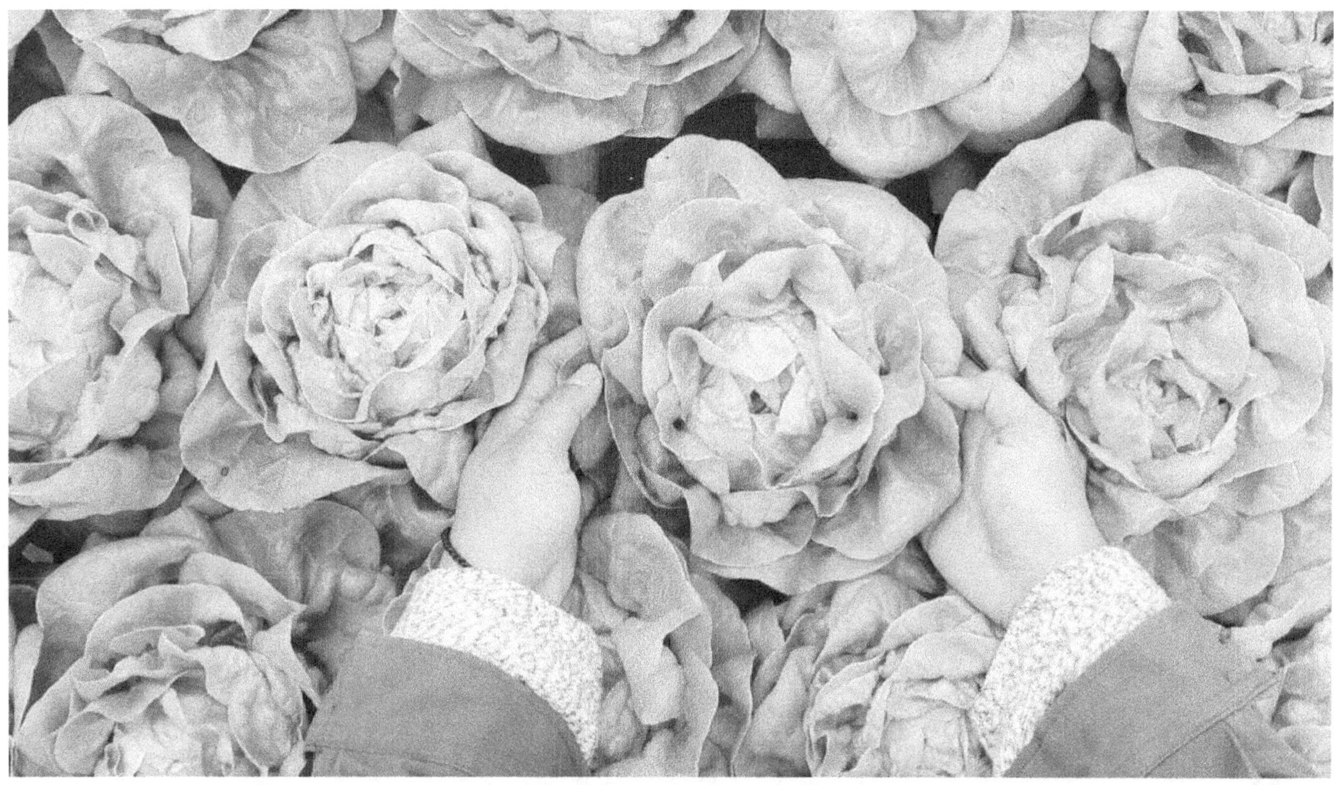

Thank you for making it to the end of the **Dr. Sebi Diet Recipes** book. 'Health is wealth,' many will say, but still, they neglect the call to give proper attention to their health for numerous reasons. Top of the list mostly is the lack of time, but when we are struck by sickness, time eventually pauses because we cannot do what we want. We fail to understand that illnesses and diseases accumulate over time, they do not just appear from nowhere. Your body must have been giving you signs, but you ignored them all.

When you start feeling tired easily, experiencing digestive distress, your allergies become more frequent, you start feeling unhealthy despite eating well, feel weak in your joints, not mentally sharp as usual, and you feel stressed out easily, etc., that is your body sending you a message. This can be likened to a car before it breaks down. It always gives off signals, like starting after several attempts, jerking, and making some weird sounds. These signals are your defense mechanism reacting to the anomalies or impending danger posed by pathogens. So, when we get these signals, we ought to act almost immediately to ensure that our body system gets back to normal.

Most times, the simple thing to do is detox, which is to rid our system of unwanted materials.